Skin Surgery and Minor Procedures

Guest Editor

FREDERICK RADKE, MD

SURGICAL CLINICS OF NORTH AMERICA

www.surgical.theclinics.com

Consulting Editor
RONALD F. MARTIN, MD

June 2009 • Volume 89 • Number 3

SAUNDERS an imprint of ELSEVIER, Inc.

W.B. SAUNDERS COMPANY

A Division of Elsevier Inc.

1600 John F. Kennedy Blvd., Suite 1800, Philadelphia, PA 19103-2899

http://www.theclinics.com

SURGICAL CLINICS OF NORTH AMERICA Volume 89, Number 3

June 2009 ISSN 0039–6109, ISBN-10: 1-4377-0546-4, ISBN-13: 978-1-4377-0546-1

Editor: Catherine Bewick

Developmental Editor: Donald Mumford

Surgical Clinics of North America (ISSN 0039–6109) is published bimonthly by Elsevier Inc., 360 Park Avenue South, New York, NY 10010-1710. Months of publication are February, April, June, August, October, and December. Business and Editorial Offices: 1600 John F. Kennedy Blvd., Suite 1800, Philadelphia, PA 19103-2899. Customer Service Office: 6277 Sea Harbor Drive, Orlando, FL 32887-4800. Periodicals postage paid at New York, NY and additional mailing offices. Subscription prices are $269.00 per year for US individuals, $432.00 per year for US institutions, $134.00 per year for US students and residents, $330.00 per year for Canadian individuals, $537.00 per year for Canadian institutions, $371.00 for international individuals, $537.00 per year for international institutions and $185.00 per year for Canadian and foreign students/residents. To receive student/resident rate, orders must be accompanied by name of affiliated institution, date of term, and the *signature* of program/residency coordinator on institution letterhead. Orders will be billed at individual rate until proof of status is received. Foreign air speed delivery is included in all *Clinics* subscription prices. All prices are subject to change without notice. POSTMASTER: Send address changes to *Surgical Clinics*, Elsevier Periodicals Customer Service, 11830 Westline Industrial Drive, St. Louis, MO 63146. **Customer Service: 1-800-654-2452 (US). From outside of the United States, call 1-314-453-7041. Fax: 1-314-453-5170. E-mail: journalscustomerservice-usa@elsevier.com (for print support), journalsonlinesupport-usa@elsevier.com (for online support).**

Reprints. For copies of 100 or more, of articles in this publication, please contact the Commercial Reprints Department, Elsevier Inc., 360 Park Avenue South, New York, New York 10010-1710. Tel. (212) 633-3812, Fax: (212) 462-1935, e-mail: reprints@elsevier.com.

The Surgical Clinics of North America is also published in Spanish by McGraw-Hill Interamericana Editores S.A., P.O. Box 5-237 06500 Mexico D.F. Mexico; and in Portuguese by Interlivros Edicoes Ltda., Rua Comandante Coelho 1085, CEP 21250, Rio de Janeiro, Brazil; and in Greek by Paschalidis Medical Publications, Athens Greece.

The Surgical Clinics of North America is covered in *MEDLINE/PubMed (Index Medicus)*, *EMBASE/Excerpta Medica*, *Current Contents/Clinical Medicine*, *Current Contents/Life Sciences*, *Science Citation Index*, and *ISI/BIOMED*.

Printed and bound by CPI Group (UK) Ltd, Croydon, CR0 4YY

Transferred to Digital Print 2011

Contributors

CONSULTING EDITOR

RONALD F. MARTIN, MD
Staff Surgeon, Marshfield Clinic, Marshfield; and Clinical Associate Professor, University of Wisconsin School of Medicine and Public Health, Madison, Wisconsin; Lieutenant Colonel, Medical Corps, United States Army Reserve

GUEST EDITOR

FREDERICK RADKE, MD
Clinical Professor, University of Vermont College of Medicine, Burlington, Vermont; and Chief, Surgical Services, Mercy Hospital, Maine Medical Center, Maine Surgical Care Group, Portland, Maine

AUTHORS

ALISHA ARORA, MD
Department of Plastic Surgery, Lahey Clinic, Burlington, Massachusetts

JOHN ATTWOOD, MD
Plastic and Hand Surgical Associates, South Portland; Director, Division of Plastic Surgery, Maine Medical Center, Portland, Maine

THOMAS H. COGBILL, MD
Program Director of Surgery Residency, Department of General and Vascular Surgery, Gundersen Lutheran Health System, La Crosse, Wisconsin

ANDREW R. DOBEN, MD
Chief Surgical Resident, Department of Surgery, Maine Medical Center, Portland, Maine

WADE W. DUNLAP, MD
Department of Surgery, Marshfield Clinic and Saint Joseph's Hospital, Marshfield, Wisconsin

VINCENT FALANGA, MD, FACP
Professor of Dermatology and Biochemistry, Department of Dermatology and Skin Surgery, Roger Williams Medical Center, Providence, Rhode Island; Department of Dermatology and Biochemistry, Boston University, Boston, Massachusetts

MARK S. GRANICK, MD
Professor and Chief, Division of Plastic Surgery, Department of Surgery, New Jersey Medical School–UMDNJ, Newark, New Jersey

SCOTT L. HANSEN, MD
Assistant Professor of Surgery (Plastic), and Chief of Hand and Microsurgery, University of California, San Francisco; and Chief of Plastic Surgery, San Francisco General Hospital, San Francisco, California

ALAN HARMATZ, MD, FACS, ASPS
Plastic and Hand Surgical Associates, South Portland, Maine

JULIO HOCHBERG, MD
Department of Surgery, Marshfield Clinic, Marshfield, Wisconsin

ERIK A. HOY, BS
Medical Student, New Jersey Medical School–UMDNJ, Newark, New Jersey

JESSE L. KAMPSHOFF, MD
Chief Resident in Surgery, Department of Medical Education, Gundersen Lutheran Medical Foundation, La Crosse, Wisconsin

SARAH KERR, MD
Dermatology Resident, Department of Dermatology, Marshfield Clinic, Marshfield, Wisconsin

JACOB M. KUSMAK, MD, PharmD
Training Director, Department of Dermatology, Marshfield Clinic, Marshfield, Wisconsin

CHARLES K. LEE, MD
Assistant Clinical Professor of Surgery (Plastic), University of California, San Francisco; and Director of Microsurgery and Wound Care, St. Mary's Medical Center, San Francisco, San Francisco, California

DOUGALD C. MACGILLIVRAY, MD, FACS
Clinical Associate Professor of Surgery, University of Vermont, Burlington, Vermont; Co-Director, Division of Surgical Oncology, Maine Medical Center; and The Maine Surgical Care Group, Portland, Maine

MICHAEL D. MARION, MD
Department of Surgery, Marshfield Clinic, Marshfield, Wisconsin

KATHLEEN M. MEYER, MD
Department of Surgery, Marshfield Clinic, Marshfield, Wisconsin

KARTIK A. PANDYA, MD
Resident Physician, Department of Surgery, Maine Medical Center, Portland, Maine

JAYMIE PANUNCIALMAN, MD
Department of Dermatology and Skin Surgery, Roger Williams Medical Center, Providence, Rhode Island

FREDERICK RADKE, MD, FACS
Clinical Professor, University of Vermont College of Medicine, Burlington, Vermont; and Chief, Surgical Services, Mercy Hospital, Maine Medical Center, Maine Surgical Care Group, Portland, Maine

ERIK J. STRATMAN, MD
Department of Dermatology, Marshfield Clinic, Marshfield, Wisconsin

PAIGE TELLER, MD
Department of Surgical Oncology, Emory University, Atlanta, Georgia

MARY TSCHOI, MD
Resident, Division of Plastic Surgery, Department of Surgery, New Jersey Medical
School–UMDNJ, Newark, New Jersey

ALFONSO L. VELASCO, MD
Department of General and Colorectal Surgery, Marshfield Clinic and Saint Joseph's
Hospital, Marshfield; Department of Surgery, Clinical Science Center, University
of Wisconsin School of Medicine and Public Health, Madison, Wisconsin

THERESE K. WHITE, MD, FACS
Plastic and Hand Surgical Associates, South Portland, Maine

Contents

The concept of wound bed preparation (WBP) heralded a new era in terms of how we treat wounds. It emphasized the difference between acute and chronic wounds, and it cemented the idea that the processes involved in the healing of acute wounds do not apply completely to the healing of chronic wounds. The arbitrary division of the normal healing process into the phases of hemostasis, inflammation, proliferation, and maturation addresses the events in acute wound healing. We have realized that the impediments to healing in chronic wounds lead to a failure to progress through these phases and are independent factors that make the chronic wound a much more complex condition. A major advance in resolving or addressing the chronic wound has been the concept of WBP. WBP allows us to address the problems of wound healing individually the presence of necrotic tissue, hypoxia, high bacterial burden, corrupt matrix, and senescent cells within the wound bed. In WBP we can optimize our therapeutic agents to accelerate endogenous healing or to increase the effectiveness of advanced therapies.

Suture application varies for different tissues, different patients, and different circumstances. The large array of new sutures, staples, tapes, and topical adhesives can make the proper choice for closure a challenge. This review of the available materials for skin closure, and their biomechanical properties, advantages, and disadvantages, creates a structure for better understanding of the limitations, indications, and numerous choices to be considered before choosing a suture material.

Open wounds, particularly around the face, often require complicated techniques for optimal closure. The approach to the closure of the complicated wound depends largely on the nature of the wound, including the location and size of the defect, the functional outcome after closure, the medical comorbidities of the patient, neighboring structures, and whether the defect is secondary to a malignancy or trauma. The goals of wound management are optimal aesthetic outcome, preservation of function, and patient satisfaction. The authors briefly review basic skin closure options and discuss use of skin flaps, particularly of the head and neck region.

> The acute wound presents a spectrum of issues that prevent its ultimate closure. These issues include host factors, etiology, anatomic location, timing, and surgical techniques to achieve successful wound closure. Basic surgical principles need to be followed to obtain stable, long-term coverage, ultimately restoring form and function. Recent advances in dressings, debridement techniques, and surgical repertoire allow the modern plastic surgeon to address any wound of any complexity. This article discusses these principles that can be applied to any wound.

> Lipomas are benign skin tumors composed of mature fat cells and are the most common subcutaneous tumors. Although many of these can be removed in the surgical clinic or minor operating room, some require more advanced preoperative planning and more complicated resection. The diagnosis, pathology, and treatment of benign tumors, and other commonly associated tumors that may require a more substantial workup and operative intervention, are discussed. Muscle and nerve biopsies are used for the diagnosis of a variety of medical problems. Although there are other genetic and biochemical markers now available that can diagnose diseases previously proven by biopsy, these surgical techniques still have appropriate uses. Although the procedures are straightforward, there are important technical issues to assist in getting the best specimen to avoid confounding disease diagnosis.

> Pilonidal disease and hidradenitis suppurativa are common problems that affect young adults. The surgical management of pilonidal disease should be tailored to the individual clinical presentation and its goal is the resolution of pilonidal disease with low recurrence and low morbidity. The clinical course of hidradenitis suppurativa is characterized by chronicity with frequent flare-ups followed by quiescent periods. Treatment for both conditions needs to be individualized to the clinical presentation.

THE CLINICS ARE NOW AVAILABLE ONLINE!

Access your subscription at:
www.theclinics.com

Foreword

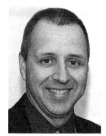

Ronald F. Martin, MD
Consulting Editor

Deep down inside—we're all superficial.
—Walter B. Goldfarb, MD

Anyone who has completed surgical training and developed a practice can attest that one learns a lot about surgery and operating in the first year of practice. For most people it is an eye-opening experience of a high order. Also, there is no such thing as a minor operation for the patient or the surgeon. Any operative procedure has the opportunity to go very well or turn out very badly. Most surgeons who have practiced for any length of time have seen plenty of examples of both types of outcomes from large, complex operations and also from operations that started out as less complex procedures.

Surgeons have a long tradition of sharing their knowledge and have written extensively about diseases that affect only a few patients and about complex procedures that even fewer surgeons will ever perform. A great source of irony in surgery is that it is not so easy to find collective writings about disorders that are far more common and about procedures that almost any general surgeon will perform someday. This collection of articles was gathered in an attempt to compile information about the more common operations surgeons perform that are discussed formally less often. For the most part the discussions involve operations that can be done in environments with limited equipment or as outpatient procedures, but some of the discussions address more complicated matters.

Although this issue addresses some of the common conditions surgeons encounter, it is worthwhile to ask why significant exposure to these common conditions is becoming more limited in current surgical education. The process of surgical education is designed to provide the surgical trainee with gradually increasing responsibility until she or he is sufficiently experienced to function safely without supervision. Overall, surgeons and surgical training programs seem to do a pretty good job in providing a mechanism for training surgeons to the degree of competence desired. There are, however, some subtle (and not so subtle) shifts in training exposure that are modifying and challenging the ability to meet those objectives.

Surg Clin N Am 89 (2009) xiii–xv
doi:10.1016/j.suc.2009.04.001
0039-6109/09/$ – see front matter

surgical.theclinics.com

The first shift that is noticeable is the relative point in training when the medical learner is exposed to direct patient care and intervention. Opportunities formerly available to junior residents and even to medical students are less likely now to occur at that level of training. There are many reasons for this shift. Among the most difficult to refute are the reasons deriving directly from the patients. Many patients are better informed consumers of medical care than in the past and are more insistent about whom they will and will not allow to participate in their care. Some of these concerns are media driven, and some probably simply reflect a shift in patient preference. The net effect remains: direct patient care is shifted to more advanced trainees and providers.

Another general shift in training programs is a change in the expectation of when along the training curve learners encounter situations that allow for personal growth. Policies are trending toward much more direct supervision, even of senior residents. There are many reasons for adopting these changes; among them are increased guidance from regulatory authorities such as the Review Committee-Surgery (RC Surgery) and the American Council for Graduate Medical Education (ACGME), increased guidance from the Joint Commission (JC), and changes in local hospital and practice policies based on concerns about litigation and risk management, and other adverse reactions.

Although many changes are attributed to these reasons, perhaps the most influential reason is simply the time available for teaching and learning. To be sure, there are still 168 hours available per week, but the allocation of these hours for clinical learning opportunities for the surgical resident has diminished and probably will continue to do so for the foreseeable future. These hour limitations have several intended consequences, but they have several unintended consequences, as well. The final net effect of these changes is uncertain at this moment, but one indisputable effect is that a new set of priorities for patient–learner interaction has developed. Gone are the days of having senior and junior residents available to participate in profoundly complex cases so that the junior resident might have more familiarity with certain operative issues when she becomes a senior resident. Also, given the present workload, senior residents are highly unlikely to perform "minor procedures" when there are "bigger" cases to cover—at least until they are within sight of residency completion; then one frequently sees a heightened and renewed interest in hernia repairs and other "intern" cases.

The fiscal pressures on staff-level surgeons are also steadily increasing and add additional impediments to incorporating and educating residents more fully in less complex procedures. "I can do this procedure alone if you have something else you need to do" is faculty code-speak for "I can get this done a lot faster by myself, and skip the beta-blockers."

The final result of the various forces involved is complicated: (1) learners encounter procedures later in training than in previous years; (2) they have fewer opportunities to participate in less complex procedures at a more advanced phase of training; and (3) they are less likely to supervise a junior learner directly in the performance of a less complex procedure with or without the presence of a staff member. In turn this system produces recent graduates who may be far more comfortable with some complex operations than they are with less complex operations performed on patients who commonly are awake and aware.

My senior partner in practice at the beginning of my career, whom I quoted above, told me, "You will have to see a lot of itchy [perineums] for every pheo you see." He was right—very right. Having a source of information that helps one deal with the more commonly seen conditions may be very valuable. To that end we appreciate the efforts of Dr. Radke and his colleagues for assembling this collection of articles. We also are appreciative of our colleagues from the *Clinics in Plastic Surgery* who prepared the informative reviews on dealing with acute wounds and skin closure techniques, which are included in this issue for our subscribers' benefit.

Ronald F. Martin, MD
Department of Surgery
Marshfield Clinic
1000 North Oak Avenue
Marshfield, WI 54449, USA

E-mail address:
martin.ronald@marshfieldclinic.org

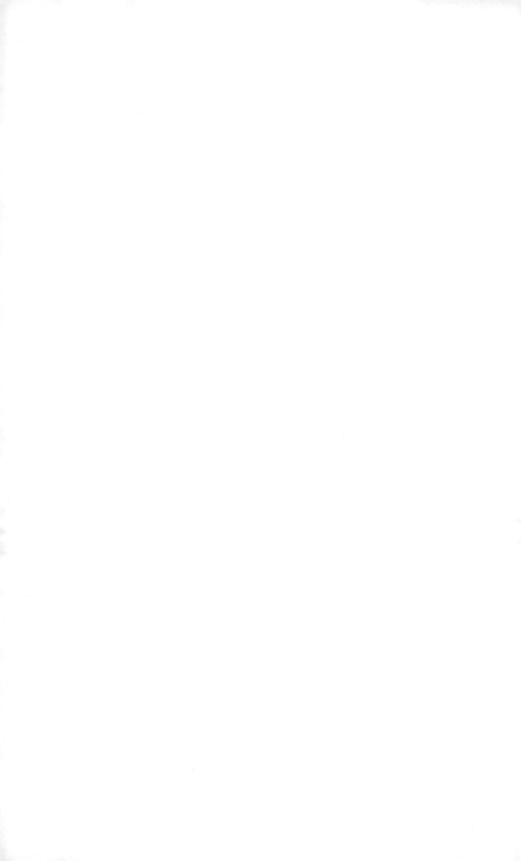

Preface

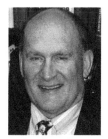

Frederick Radke, MD
Guest Editor

This issue of the *Surgical Clinics of North America* is designed to give the readers a summary of basic knowledge of problems of the skin and subcutaneous tissues. The authors have prepared a series of articles ranging from the basic science of wound healing to the clinically frustrating problems of pilonidal disease.

I thank each of the authors for their efforts. In addition, I would like to thank the strength of this series: Ronald Martin, MD, and Catherine Bewick of Elsevier. They were generous with their time, patience, and advice.

We hope that these articles will inspire the readers. A number of the authors from Maine Medical Center have been inspired in this field by the efforts and example of Dr. Jean Labelle. We would like to show our appreciation by dedicating this issue to him.

Frederick Radke, MD
Maine Medical Center
22 Bramhall Street
Portland, ME 04192, USA

E-mail address: radkef@mmc.org

Surg Clin N Am 89 (2009) xvii
doi:10.1016/j.suc.2009.04.002
0039-6109/09/$ – see front matter

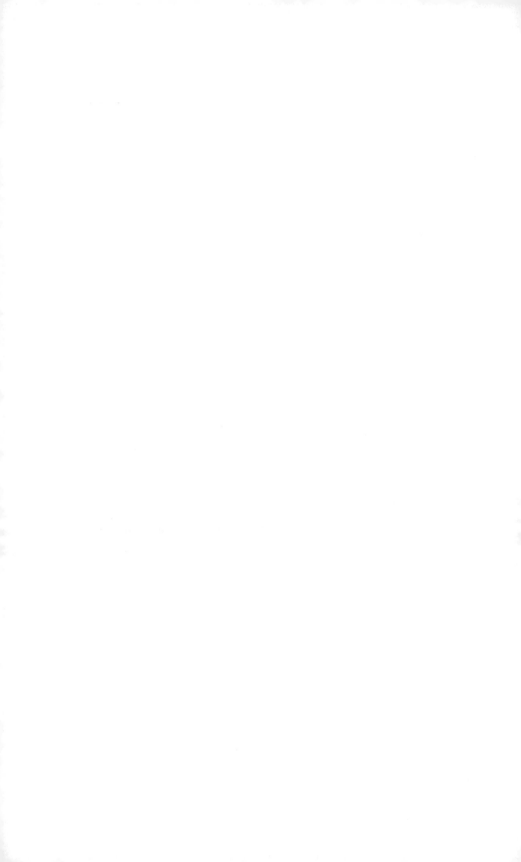

Dermatology for the General Surgeon

Sarah Kerr, MD, Jacob M. Kusmak, MD, PharmD, Erik J. Stratman, MD*

KEYWORDS

- Atopic dermatitis • Dermatology for surgeon • Intertrigo
- Psoriasis • Surgical infection risk

In addition to encountering the skin with nearly every procedure, the surgeon will also likely experience skin-related conundrums, concerns, and associated conditions in the preoperative, perioperative, or postoperative periods. These occasionally lead to dermatologic consultation. On review of consultative requests from surgeons at our institution over a 10-year period, the consultation requests can be summarized into key areas: (1) Can the patient's skin disease be cleared by the operative date and, if not, can the procedure safely occur without increased risk of postoperative complications from infection? (2) Do skin conditions occurring outside the surgical field affect postoperative risk of infection? (3) Do the patient's cutaneous findings provide clues to the underlying surgical condition? (4) Which perioperative or postoperative drug caused a drug exanthem or contact dermatitis?

In this review, these concerns are addressed using best available evidence. The first section provides the surgeon with recommendations for the more common cutaneous diseases encountered in the preoperative period. In the second section, preoperative assessment of dermatologic therapies is discussed. A few key categories are reviewed, including a variety of common topical medications, biologic treatments, and oral retinoids. The third section highlights cutaneous associations of operable visceral disease, including inflammatory bowel disease (IBD), familial cancer syndromes, and syndromes associated with internal hemorrhage. In the fourth section, consideration is given to skin conditions arising in the postoperative period, including morbilliform drug eruptions, allergic contact dermatitis, and skin conditions resulting from surgical procedures. Although not exhaustive, the goal of this article is to provide dermatologic considerations pertinent to the evaluation and care of a surgical patient. Surgical management of cutaneous malignancies and management of postoperative wound infections are not addressed.

Department of Dermatology, Marshfield Clinic, 1000 North Oak Avenue (3P2), Marshfield, WI 54449, USA
* Corresponding author.
E-mail address: stratman.erik@marshfieldclinic.org (E.J. Stratman).

Surg Clin N Am 89 (2009) 563–586
doi:10.1016/j.suc.2009.02.004
0039-6109/09/$ – see front matter © 2009 Elsevier Inc. All rights reserved.
surgical.theclinics.com

PREOPERATIVE CONSIDERATIONS AND MANAGEMENT OF COMMON SKIN DISEASE

Several chronic skin conditions occur in the general population. Three common conditions that trigger a consultative request or inquiry are psoriasis, atopic dermatitis, and intertrigo. Each is discussed in a surgical context.

Psoriasis

As the prevalence of psoriasis is 1% to 5% in the general population in the United States, it is likely that the surgeon will encounter patients with this disease.[1] Psoriasis is a polygenic, chronic, relapsing, T cell mediated inflammatory skin disease with many triggering factors, including trauma, infection, and medications. The classic clinical presentation is thick, silvery-scaled, sharply defined, pink plaques occurring on the scalp, elbows, and knees. However, in chronic plaque-type psoriasis, lesions can occur anywhere. Clinical presentations can be variable. In addition to chronic plaque-type, guttate (droplike showers of small psoriasis lesions over the body, typically poststreptococcal), erythrodermic (psoriasis affecting the entire skin surface), inverse (psoriasis affecting principally the body folds, appearing more glazed red, rather than silvery-scaled), and pustular psoriasis exist. Pertinent to the surgeon operating on a patient with psoriasis is the disease-specific isomorphic response, or Kœbner phenomenon, in which psoriatic lesions may appear at sites of injury, including scratches, burns, and surgical incisions (**Fig. 1**).[2]

Patients with psoriasis have higher streptococcal and staphylococcal skin carriage rates compared with normal controls.[3–5] Despite this, there is evidence that as long as proper skin preparation for surgical procedures is performed, there is no higher incidence of skin infection and healing time,[6,7] with the possible exception of patients with psoriatic arthritis undergoing total knee arthroplasty.[8] Although high-level (type A) evidence is lacking on assessment of infection risk following surgery on the patient with psoriasis, the assessment of dermatologists is that the infection risk is low.[3]

Given the paucity of definitive data, during the weeks preceding elective surgery, it is reasonable to treat aggressively any psoriasis lesions located within the planned surgical field. If the psoriasis affecting the surgical field is <10% to 15% of the total body surface area, topical therapy with clobetasol ointment applied 1 to 2 times daily to the affected skin is the treatment of choice in the weeks preceding surgery. If time to operation is <4 to 6 weeks, the efficacy of clobetasol can be increased by occluding the area with telfa or plastic wrap after topical steroid application. If the eruption

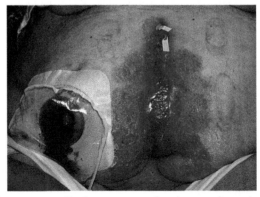

Fig. 1. Kœbner phenomenon. Erythematous, scaly plaque of psoriasis surrounding an abdominal wound in a surgical patient. (*Courtesy of* E.J. Stratman, MD, Marshfield, WI.)

clears, then the patient should discontinue clobetasol. If the psoriasis within a surgical field is >15% body surface area, clobetasol can still be used, but patient adherence to the regimen often drops. Systemic treatments may be entertained at that point. Cyclosporine typically leads to rapid improvement of psoriasis. Ultraviolet treatment with narrow-band (310–313 nm) ultraviolet B (UVB) therapy also offers a quick response but without as many immunosuppressive effects as cyclosporine. Unfortunately, narrow-band UVB usually requires access to a dermatology office and in-office treatments 3 times weekly. If the preoperative interval is insufficient to lead to effective treatment of surgical field psoriasis, preoperative antibiotic should be chosen with adequate gram-positive coverage.

Atopic Dermatitis

Atopic dermatitis is a chronic, relapsing form of eczema that occurs at any age, affecting up to 20% of the population in the United States.[9] This condition usually presents before the age of 5, and may be associated with allergic rhinitis and asthma.[9] Classic clinical manifestations include focally crusted, lichenified, scaly erythematous patches occurring in symmetric locations, often including the popliteal and antecubital fossae, hands, head, and neck (**Fig. 2**A, B). Like psoriasis, atopic dermatitis can occur anywhere on the skin surface. Lesions of atopic dermatitis tend to be more pruritic and less sharply defined than psoriasis.

Patients with atopic dermatitis have a high *Staphylococcus aureus* and beta-hemolytic streptococcus carriage rate in lesional and nonlesional skin.[10,11] Secondary infections are associated with atopic dermatitis, especially if the disease is not well managed.[9,11] Surface bacteria and viruses flourish if the skin barrier function is defective. Some pathogenic bacteria, through the actions of superantigens, trigger a worsening of the atopic flare.[12] Due to infection risk, the surgeon should postpone elective surgery rather than incise through actively inflamed dermatitis.[13] Lesional

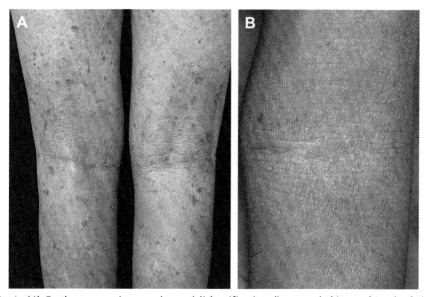

Fig. 2. (*A*) Erythema, erosions, scale, and lichenification (increased skin markings) of the popliteal fossae. (*B*) Confluent erythema and lichenification in the antecubital fossa. (*Courtesy of* E.J. Stratman, MD, Marshfield, WI.)

bacterial counts decrease dramatically if therapies targeting dermatitis are applied.[14] A safe preoperative regimen involves daily use of a modified Dakin's solution consisting of one fourth cup of household bleach in a bathtub of water or 0.25% bleach in sterile water irrigation solution (2.5 mL/1,000 mL sterile water, available as a commercial product). In adults, midpotency topical steroids such as triamcinolone 0.1% ointment are appropriate first line agents. In general, ointments tend to sting less compared with creams or lotions when applied to atopic skin.

Intertrigo

Intertrigo is a superficial inflammatory dermatitis occurring most often in areas where two skin surfaces are in contact, making the environment moist, warm, and easily macerated. Intertrigo often occurs in obese patients and most often occurs in the infrapannus, inframammary, gluteal, and inguinal folds. It appears bright red and glazed, sometimes with superficial erosions or satellite lesions. Candida should be considered if satellite papules are present. Fine scales can be present at the periphery of the affected skin, and sometimes small, round, scaly, red satellite lesions can be found (**Fig. 3**). Secondary skin infections can occur with intertrigo, including candida, dermatophyte, staphylococcus, streptococcus, pseudomonas, or corynebacteria. Because intertrigo harbors microorganisms, surgical incisions through these areas should be avoided if at all possible.[15,16]

Because of the combination of inflammation and the presence of pathogenic microorganisms, a combined topical approach is best if clearing intertrigo is desirable before surgery. Mixing a mild topical steroid (2.5% hydrocortisone or desonide 0.05% ointment) in equal parts with a broad spectrum antimicrobial with good antiyeast coverage (iodoquinol or econazole) leads to control of most intertrigo if applied twice daily and combined with a cornstarch-free powder regimen to affected areas. Physical barriers to minimize skin-on-skin irritation can also be of benefit. These include cotton cloth, gauze, or zinc oxide paste or ointment applied daily. Up to 2 weeks of treatment is typically needed before the microorganism count is negligible. If the surgical field is distant to this affected field, surgery need not be postponed.

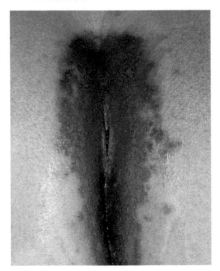

Fig. 3. Confluent bright erythema with erythematous satellite papules and slight fissuring in the gluteal cleft. (*Courtesy of* Marshfield Clinic Department, Marshfield, WI.)

Viral Skin Diseases

The surgeon will likely encounter several viral skin diseases within or near the surgical field, including warts, molluscum, herpes simplex (types I or II), and herpes zoster. Although warts and molluscum could spread to injured skin or any vigorously scrubbed areas, these do not have the potential to significantly impact intraoperative or postoperative outcomes. Surgical scrubs that contain povidone iodine, chlorhexidine gluconate, or benzalkonium chloride inactivate most viruses.[17]

Herpes simplex virus (HSV) types I and II are difficult to distinguish clinically without the assistance of laboratory studies. Both present as 1- to 4-mm clustered vesicles (**Fig. 4**A), which progressively break down to shallow, grouped erosions and ulcers (see **Fig. 4**B). Lesions are predominantly distributed in mucocutaneous areas of the body, including the oral mucosae and genital regions, but can occur anywhere.

Herpes zoster is a reactivation of the varicella zoster virus (VZV), the cause of chickenpox. After primary infection with VZV, the virus lies dormant in the dorsal root ganglia of the spine or ganglia of the cranial nerves (most common). Emotional or physical stress most commonly triggers reactivation, which classically follows a unilateral dermatomal distribution. Although typically limited in severity, in immunocompromised patients, herpes zoster can disseminate to the visceral organs, leading to life-threatening hemorrhagic necrosis of the pancreas, liver, lung, or bowel.[18]

Limited research has addressed whether it is appropriate to perform an operation in a patient with active HSV1, HSV2, or VZV skin disease. If surgery is indicated in a patient with active HSV or zoster skin lesions, perioperative antiviral medication should be given expeditiously. If discovered at the time of surgery, intravenous acyclovir at dosage appropriate for the patient's size and renal function can be given. If the timing of surgery allows oral therapy, valacyclovir has higher oral absorption than its parent drug, acyclovir. For recurrent HSV, valacyclovir 2000 mg, twice daily for 1 day is a rapid 1-day treatment regimen. Valacyclovir 1000 mg 3 times daily for 7 days is the regimen of choice for herpes zoster. If possible, the lesions should be left intact, as the virus is found at the base of the vesicle. Once lesions are crusted, the patient is no longer considered infectious.

PREOPERATIVE ASSESSMENT OF DERMATOLOGIC THERAPIES

In the preoperative period, surgeons are accountable for assessing current patient medications that may impact the surgical outcome. Medications for dermatologic conditions are numerous. These medications include, but are not limited to, topical,

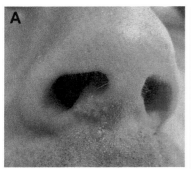 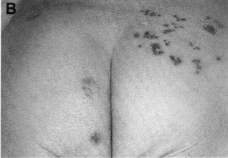

Fig. 4. (A) Clustered vesicles on an erythematous base in active herpes simplex. (B) Herpetic groups of punched out, shallow crusted erosions in resolving herpes simplex. (*Courtesy of* E.J. Stratman, MD, Marshfield, WI.)

oral, injectable, and intravenous products, including newer biologic treatments. A few key categories are reviewed, including a variety of common topical medications, oral retinoids, and biologic treatments.

Topical Corticosteroids

For the 3 common skin conditions discussed earlier, recommendations for preoperative treatment include prescription of topical steroids. Pertinent local effects of topical steroids on skin include epidermal atrophy, delayed re-epithelialization, reduced collagen and ground substance formation, and impaired angiogenesis.[19–21] Delayed wound healing is theoretically possible if the surgical site includes an area under steroid treatment, especially if ultrapotent steroids (clobetasol, halobetasol, augmented betamethasone dipropionate) are in use, and if the treatment time has exceeded 2 to 4 weeks. Minimal impact on wound healing can be expected if topical steroids are used within the surgical field in the 2 weeks before surgery. Direct application of topical steroids to a wound is not recommended due to the delay in healing. Systemic absorption from topical steroid application is possible, but typically is insignificant. Hypothalamic-pituitary axis suppression is not likely to be significant in the adult. If it occurs, it is mainly due to chronic therapy over large surface areas using high-potency products.

Calcineurin Inhibitors

Tacrolimus and pimecrolimus represent a class of topical immunomodulators used to treat a variety of inflammatory dermatologic disorders. These topicals suppress the release of proinflammatory cytokines and prevent T cell activation in the skin. These products have been approved by the US Food and Drug Administration for use in atopic dermatitis, and are used in some cases of inverse psoriasis, seborrheic dermatitis, and intertrigo. Despite a black-box warning for questions about malignancy risk with repeated use, the side effect profiles for calcineurin inhibitors are favorable.[22–24] Unlike topical steroids, neither of these agents has been associated with skin atrophy and they do not affect the collagen synthesis processes.[23,24] Additionally, no adverse effect on wound healing has been reported, and these medications are not associated with an increase in bacterial or viral infections, with the possible exception of varicella in childhood.[23,24] The perioperative use of calcineurin inhibitors should be safe.

Systemic Retinoids

Isotretinoin and acitretin are oral retinoid therapies that have a significant impact on dermatologic diseases, including scarring acne (isotretinoin) and psoriasis (acitretin). Both are reported to have a negative impact on wound healing. Initial animal studies involving mice and guinea pigs showed a possible delay in wound healing involving isotretinoin.[25,26] However, a study of acitretin on humans in 2004 evaluated the perioperative risks with organ transplant recipients undergoing skin surgery and revealed that acitretin does not increase the risk of wound-healing complications in this patient population.[27] Nonetheless, most patients are typically counseled to delay elective procedures until at least 1 month after concluding oral retinoids.

Biologic Treatments

Another class of medications used in the treatment of psoriasis, psoriatic arthritis, and other dermatologic diseases is the biologic response modifiers. Medications in this class work by a variety of specific molecular mechanisms that target proteins, antibodies, or cytokines. The biologic medications include abatacept, adalimumab, alefacept, efalizumab, etanercept, and infliximab.[1,28] These treatments have good efficacy and are well tolerated by patients, even though they may have variable side effects. In particular, the use of these medications has been associated with a high risk of infection.[1] Thus, perioperative therapy modification is recommended.[29] For these biologic agents, general recommendations are to discontinue the medication 1 week before surgery and restart 1 to 2 weeks after surgery. The strongest evidence for these recommendations is with etanercept and adalimumab.

SKIN FINDINGS WITH BOWEL DISEASE, MALIGNANCY SYNDROMES AND VASCULAR SYNDROMES

There are several diseases in which cutaneous manifestations or associated skin findings observed at the time of initial surgical consultation or evaluation may help to identify the underlying cause of the surgical condition. Simple examples include jaundice with scleral icterus in the setting of a biliary tree obstruction, or a Sister Mary Joseph nodule in the setting of metastatic adenocarcinoma. This section explores the skin manifestations of IBD, familial cancer syndromes, and genetic causes of acute gastrointestinal bleeding, in an attempt to clinically aid the surgeon in diagnostic preparation for surgery or other intervention.

Skin Findings Associated with IBD

The term "inflammatory bowel disease" encompasses a group of conditions including Crohn disease and ulcerative colitis. There are several extra-intestinal manifestations associated with IBD, and the 3 most commonly affected organ systems are the muco-cutaneous, musculoskeletal, and ocular systems.[30] Reports on the prevalence of extra-intestinal manifestations vary widely, likely because of variances in how these manifestations are defined.[30,31] Further discussion is limited to mucocutaneous findings, which include metastatic cutaneous Crohn disease, pyoderma gangrenosum, erythema nodosum, aphthous ulcers, and Sweet syndrome.

The most frequent cutaneous manifestations of Crohn disease are perianal fissures and fistulae, and either manifestation may be the presenting sign. Around 7% of patients have perianal disease at the time of diagnosis, with 45% of patients experiencing it at some time during the disease course.[31]

Cutaneous or metastatic Crohn should only be considered if granulomatous lesions occur at a site remote from the gastrointestinal tract.[31] Although cutaneous Crohn disease is rare, two thirds of children and one half of adult patients with cutaneous Crohn disease have involvement of the genitalia. Erythema and edema of the labia or scrotum may be the first signs of this disease process.[32] Commonly affected extra-genital sites include intertriginous areas and the lower extremities,[31] although any other area may be involved.[30] The clinical appearance of lesions varies widely. Granulomatous papules, erythematous plaques, draining sinuses, ulcers with undermined borders, fissures, or even vegetations may be seen and can lead to scarring (**Fig. 5**). Cutaneous activity is generally unrelated to bowel inflammation. Histopathology is similar to that of intestinal lesions and consists of noncaseating granulomas in the dermis that may extend to subcutaneous fat.[31] Topical tacrolimus 0.1% ointment may lead to improvement of fissures, papules, and plaques.[33,34] Otherwise the systemic therapies used in intestinal Crohn disease can benefit most cutaneous manifestations.

Erythema nodosum is a form of panniculitis that presents as erythematous, tender nodules, commonly found on the anterior shins (**Fig. 6**). If associated with IBD, erythema nodosum is usually seen within the first 2 years of IBD symptoms. Prevalence of erythema nodosum in these patients varies from 3% to 20%.[31] Lesions

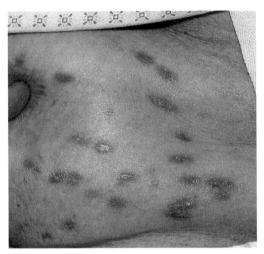

Fig. 5. Multiple reddish brown granulomatous lesions of cutaneous Crohn disease. (*Courtesy of* E.J. Stratman, MD, Marshfield, WI.)

may occur on the thighs and arms, and rarely on the trunk, face, and neck. The lesions erupt acutely, may be bilateral, and do not ulcerate or scar. Erythema nodosum can also be associated with streptococcal infections, sarcoidosis, coccidioidomycosis, systemic medications, pregnancy, and other diseases.[35] If the cutaneous lesions occur in conjunction with IBD, their course usually corresponds with gastrointestinal disease activity.[30,31] The therapeutic ladder for erythema nodosum includes

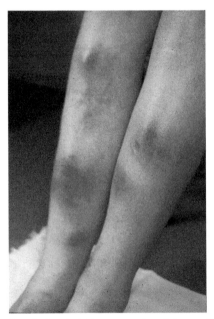

Fig. 6. Multiple erythematous indurated plaques and nodules on the anterior shins consistent with erythema nodosum. (*Courtesy of* Marshfield Clinic Department, Marshfield, WI.)

nonsteroidal antiinflammatory agents, a supersaturated solution of potassium iodide, or systemic glucocorticoids for severe, recalcitrant disease.

Oral aphthae are common with up to 20% of the general population affected. If 3 or more oral aphthae (**Fig. 7**) or oral and genital aphthae are present most of the time, the diagnosis of IBD must be entertained, along with Behçet's disease, vitamin deficiencies, human immunodeficiency virus, and others.[36] Deficiencies of iron, folic acid, and vitamin B12 should not be overlooked, and supplementation may lead to improvement of the aphthae.[36] Other possible oral manifestations of IBD include cobblestoning of the buccal mucosa, angular cheilitis, oral edema, gingival hyperplasia or nodules, and indurated fissuring of the lower lip.[37]

Pyoderma gangrenosum is a recurrent neutrophilic dermatosis that can be associated with a wide variety of underlying systemic diseases, including IBD, rheumatologic, hepatic, or hematologic disease, visceral carcinoma, human immunodeficiency virus, and sarcoidosis.[38] Among patients with pyoderma gangrenosum, 50% to 75% will have an identifiable underlying disease, and up to 2% of patients with IBD will develop pyoderma gangrenosum. As with most other extra-intestinal manifestations of IBD, the activity of cutaneous disease does not correlate with bowel inflammation. There are 4 forms of pyoderma gangrenosum: ulcerative, pustular, bullous, and vegetative.[38,39] Pyostomatitis vegetans is another condition similar to pyoderma gangrenosum that can affect the labial and buccal mucosa of patients with IBD.[38]

Ulcerative pyoderma gangrenosum is considered the classic form of pyoderma gangrenosum. Lesions are typically solitary, and usually start as small, often perifollicular, pustules and rapidly expand to produce ulcers with irregular undermined borders (**Fig. 8**). Pathergy, or lesion development at a site of minor trauma, is demonstrated in up to 50% of cases.[39] Because of pathergy, debridement or other surgical intervention including skin grafting is not indicated and may cause disease progression. Lesions are usually painful, occurring most commonly on the lower extremities, but can occur anywhere.[38,39] In children, lesions are of similar morphology but are distributed more commonly on the head, neck, and genital area.[38] Scarring is common.[38,39] Similar to ulcerative pyoderma gangrenosum, peristomal pyoderma gangrenosum accounts for about 15% of all pyoderma gangrenosum cases. Peristomal pyoderma gangrenosum occurs in the skin near or adjacent to the stoma following bowel surgery. It is painful and may interfere greatly with the function and adhesion of the stoma bag. Concurrent irritant dermatitis may also become problematic due to bag contents coming into contact with skin.[39]

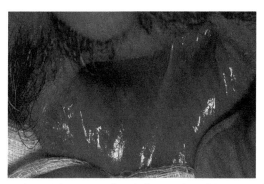

Fig. 7. Oral aphthous ulcer with surrounding inflammation. (*Courtesy of* Marshfield Clinic Department, Marshfield, WI.)

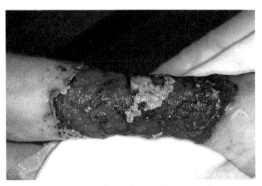

Fig. 8. Large pyoderma gangrenosum ulceration with necrotic center and irregular, violaceous, undermined border. (*Courtesy of* Marshfield Clinic Department, Marshfield, WI.)

Sweet syndrome is another neutrophilic dermatosis associated with IBD, hematologic or visceral malignancies, medications, and pregnancy. Classic Sweet syndrome presents clinically as tender, erythematous to violaceous edematous papules, plaques, and nodules that may have a vesicular or pseudovesicular appearance (**Fig. 9**).[40] These lesions are distributed asymmetrically, most commonly on the face, upper extremities, and neck, but can occur anywhere and usually resolve without scarring. Patients can be systemically ill with fever, malaise, arthralgias, myalgias, and headache. An elevated neutrophil count is common. These symptoms may precede the cutaneous eruption by a period of days or weeks.

About 20% of persons with Sweet syndrome will have an underlying malignancy, with men and women equally affected. In other causes, women are more likely affected. In other causes, there is a predominance in women. Treatment of the underlying malignancy or removal of the causative medication will usually result in resolution of the cutaneous lesions.[40] The average age of onset is 30 to 60 years. Despite fevers and lesions resembling cellulitis or erysipelas, the lesions of Sweet syndrome are sterile and do not present an increased risk for postoperative infection. Multiple treatments have been described for Sweet syndrome, including topical, intralesional, and systemic steroids, potassium iodide, dapsone, colchicine, and nonsteroidal antiinflammatory agents, with prednisone considered first-line therapy in most cases requiring treatment.[40]

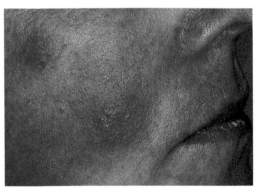

Fig. 9. Juicy, erythematous plaques with pseudovesicular appearance in a patient with Sweet syndrome. (*Courtesy of* E.J. Stratman, MD, Marshfield, WI.)

With the exception of cutaneous Crohn disease, the mucocutaneous diseases discussed earlier may be seen in association with diseases other than IBD. If associated with IBD, activity of skin lesions does not typically correlate with bowel disease activity.

Familial Cancer Syndromes

Some internal malignancies requiring surgery will be part of a larger familial cancer syndrome that may have cutaneous manifestations. Cutaneous clues may assist in timely preoperative diagnosis and in the selection of further investigations that may lead to diagnosis of the syndrome, allowing more timely notification and screening of family and, if needed, the use of appropriate surveillance examinations. Commercial tests are available for most of the diseases described in this section for testing patients and their family members. Web sites with such test information are available and they are updated regularly as testing advances occur.[41]

Peutz-Jeghers Syndrome (OMIM 175200)

Peutz-Jeghers syndrome is an autosomal dominant disease marked by gastrointestinal hamartomatous polyps and pigmented macules on mucocutaneous surfaces. Spontaneous mutations account for 50% of cases,[42] and reported incidence varies widely ranging from 1 in 50,000 to 1 in 200,000. The polyps in Peutz-Jeghers syndrome are true hamartomas, occurring most commonly in the small intestine, but may also be seen in the colon and stomach. Most patients are diagnosed due to gastrointestinal problems, including obstruction, intussusception, abdominal pain, blood in the stool, or even anal extrusion of a polyp. Only 13% of patients are diagnosed due to the characteristic melanin pigmentation. The pigmented macules are present at birth or appear during infancy, and are usually distributed around the mouth, on the lip vermillion, palate, tongue, and buccal mucosa (**Fig. 10**). Periorbital pigmented macules also occur, and lesions may be seen on the hands and feet.[43] The brown macules may fade with age, but those on the buccal mucosa usually remain. Freckles, or ephelides, are not found on the buccal mucosa and are rarely distributed in a dense manner around the nose or mouth. A solitary brown macule on the lip vermillion, referred to as a labial melanotic macule, is not associated with the syndrome. Reported malignancies include esophageal, stomach, pancreatic, intestinal, colon, breast, ovarian, uterine, cervical, and lung cancers.[43,44]

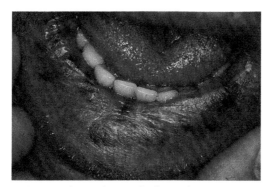

Fig. 10. Characteristic pigmented macules on the lower lip in a patient with Peutz-Jeghers syndrome. (*Courtesy of* E.J. Stratman, MD, Marshfield, WI.)

Gardner Syndrome (OMIM 175100)

Caused by a germline mutation in the APC gene on chromosome 5q21, Gardner syndrome is an autosomal dominant disease marked by intestinal polyposis with an almost certain progression to colon cancer if prophylactic colectomy is not performed. Cutaneous lesions may precede the discovery of colon polyps and consist of epidermoid cysts, which are seen in 35% of cases. Cysts may first appear in the young child and are most commonly found on the scalp, face, and trunk (**Fig. 11**). Over time they tend to increase in size and number. Other cutaneous manifestations of Gardner syndrome include leiomyomas, lipomas, and fibromas.[45] Osteomas, which occur commonly in the mandible, affect 80% of persons with Gardner syndrome. Dental abnormalities, such as impacted or supranummary teeth, and congenital hyperplasia of the retinal pigment epithelium may also be present.[45]

Muir-Torre Syndrome (OMIM 158320)

Muir-Torre syndrome was first described in 1967[46] and is associated with multiple types of malignancies, of which colorectal cancer is the most common. Other associated cancers include those arising in the endometrium, ovary, bladder, kidney, ureter, breast, and upper gastrointestinal tract. Hematological malignancies and tumors of the parotid gland and larynx have also been reported.[47] This is an autosomal dominant syndrome caused by a mutation in the *MSH2* DNA mismatch repair gene. Mutations in the *MLH1* gene have also been reported. Median age at diagnosis is 55 years, and 28% to 41% of patients have cutaneous findings at the time of diagnosis.[47,48]

The cutaneous lesions seen in Muir-Torre syndrome are sebaceous neoplasms, including sebaceous adenomas, epitheliomas, basal cell carcinomas with sebaceous differentiation, and sebaceous carcinomas. Keratoacanthomas should be considered a marker only if the patient has two or more visceral malignancies and multiple lesions, as well as a family history of the syndrome, or if the keratoacanthoma demonstrates sebaceous differentiation.[47] Sebaceous adenomas are benign tumors that appear clinically as yellow papules or nodules. Up to 70% occur on the head and neck. Sebaceous epitheliomas are difficult to distinguish clinically and differ histologically from the adenoma in the quantity of undifferentiated sebaceous cells (adenomas have

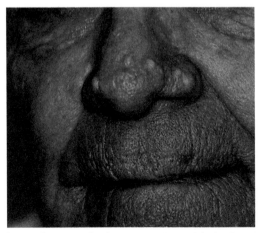

Fig. 11. Multiple epidermoid cysts on the face in a patient with Gardner syndrome. (*Courtesy of* E.J. Stratman, MD, Marshfield, WI.)

more than epitheliomas). Sebaceous carcinoma is a malignant neoplasm that occurs most commonly on the eyelid but may occur elsewhere. Patients are often diagnosed with conjunctivitis, carbuncles, or chalazia before biopsy. Keratoacanthomas present as a crateriform nodule that grows rapidly and may have a central keratotic plug.[48] Sebaceous hyperplasia, commonly occurring as small, flesh-colored to yellow-orange multilobulated papules, is not an associated finding. The nevus sebaceus of Jadassohn is not related to Muir-Torre syndrome.[47,48]

Cowden Disease (OMIM 158350)

Cowden disease is an autosomal dominant disorder characterized by mucocutaneous neoplasia, gastrointestinal tract hamartomas, breast carcinoma, and thyroid carcinoma.[49] A germline mutation in the tumor suppressor gene *PTEN* is responsible for Cowden disease. The reported incidence is 1 in 200,000, and although most patients first note cutaneous signs in their teens or twenties, age at diagnosis ranges from 13 to 65 years.[50] Skin and mucosal lesions, which occur in almost 100% of persons with Cowden disease, most commonly consist of trichilemmomas and papillomatous papules. Trichilemmomas are benign hamartomatous growths derived from the outer root sheath of the hair follicle.[49] Clinically, they appear as small, flesh-colored warty papules similar to common warts and are generally distributed more centrally around the eyes, nose, mouth, chin, and sometimes on the hands, and feet (**Fig. 12**A). Lesions also occur on the oral mucosa, giving it a cobblestoned appearance (see **Fig. 12**B).[49,51] Other cutaneous signs include acral keratoses which appear as small pits in the palms or soles, sclerotic fibromas, lipomas, hemangiomas, lentigines, and xanthomas.[50,52]

The most common malignancy in the setting of Cowden disease is adenocarcinoma of the breast, occurring in 25% to 50% of patients.[49,50] Thyroid cancer is the second most common cancer. Other associated malignancies include renal carcinoma, endometrial carcinoma, and glial tumors. Other manifestations of Cowden disease include

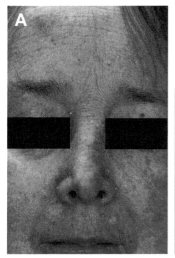
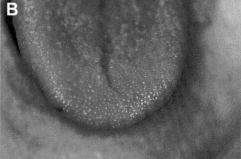

Fig. 12. (*A*) Pink and flesh-colored warty papules on the central face of a patient with Cowden disease. (*B*) Papillomatous papules give the tongue a cobblestoned appearance in Cowden disease. (*Courtesy of* E.J. Stratman, MD, Marshfield, WI.)

benign breast, thyroid, and uterine neoplasms, cerebellar enlargement, macroce-phaly, and abnormalities of the palate, mandible, and maxilla.[49–51]

Birt-Hogg-Dubé (OMIM 135150)

Young persons with lung cysts or a history of spontaneous pneumothorax or patients with renal tumors, particularly chromophobe or oncocytic carcinomas, along with multiple cutaneous papules on the face or neck should prompt consideration of Birt-Hogg-Dubé (BHD) syndrome. The skin lesions of BHD include fibrofolliculomas, trichodiscomas, and less diagnostic findings, including acrochordons and angiofibro-mas.[53,54] Fibrofolliculomas and trichodiscomas are uncommon outside the setting of this syndrome, and present as flesh-colored to ivory, smooth, discrete, firm papules, usually 2 to 4 mm in size (**Fig. 13**A, B), found most often on the forehead, nose, and cheeks. Acrochordons, which appear as soft, pedunculated light tan to brown papules, are seen more commonly in flexural areas.[55] Angiofibromas appear clinically similar to fibrofolliculomas; however, angiofibromas are more often pink or telangiec-tatic.[54] Colonic polyps and colon cancer are not associated manifestations, a common misconception in earlier descriptions of the disease.[53,55] A mutation in the BHD tumor suppressor gene that encodes folliculin leads to the pathology seen in the skin, lung, and kidney.[54]

Due to the increased risk of renal tumors, abdominal computed tomography or renal ultrasound is recommended at the time of diagnosis, with continued surveillance every 3 to 5 years. Routine health care of all siblings should be encouraged, with skin biopsy and renal diagnostics, as appropriate.[55]

Vascular Abnormalities

The surgeon is often required to evaluate the patient with an acute gastrointestinal bleed. Certain skin findings can provide clues for syndromic causes for such hemor-rhage, which might help in the initial approach to such patients and lead to appropriate screening procedures for relatives.

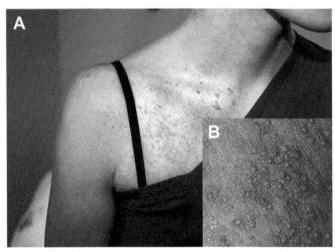

Fig. 13. (A) Multiple fibrofolliculomas in a patient with Birt-Hogg-Dubé syndrome. (B) Close-up of the flesh-colored, firm, smooth, domed papules. (Courtesy of E.J. Stratman, MD, Marshfield, WI.)

Hereditary Hemorrhagic Telangiectasia (OMIM 187300)

Hereditary hemorrhagic telangiectasia (HHT), or Osler-Weber-Rendu, is an autosomal dominant disorder caused by mutations of either the endoglin or *ALK-1* gene with a reported prevalence of 1 in 5,000 to 1 in 10,000.[56,57] It is characterized by mucocutaneous telangiectasias, arteriovenous malformations, and telangiectasia of the gastrointestinal tract, and arteriovenous malformations of the lung, liver, and central nervous system.[56] Recurrent epistaxis due to telangiectasia of the nasal mucosa is usually the first sign, and mat telangiectasias of the face, lips, tongue, buccal mucosa, upper extremities, and nail beds usually follow within 5 to 30 years (**Fig. 14**).[57,58] Telangiectasias of the gastrointestinal mucosa may also occur, most commonly in the stomach and duodenum. These and gastrointestinal arteriovenous malformations are a cause of significant bleeding in about 16% of persons with HHT.[58] Although the mucocutaneous telangiectasias are commonly of cosmetic concern, arteriovenous malformations in the lung, liver, and central nervous system may lead to serious consequences, including respiratory complications, stroke, emboli, seizure, and hemorrhage. The diagnosis of HHT is established if any three of the following criteria are met: (1) spontaneous recurrent nosebleeds; (2) mucocutaneous telangiectasia in characteristic distribution; (3) visceral lesions including arteriovenous malformations of the lung, liver, gastrointestinal tract, or central nervous system; or (4) first degree relative with HHT. If two of the criteria are met, the diagnosis of HHT must be suspected.[58]

Blue Rubber Bleb Nevus Syndrome (OMIM 112200)

Before 2004, fewer than 150 cases of blue rubber bleb nevus syndrome (BRBNS) were reported. Similar to HHT, BRBNS is a disease with mucocutaneous and visceral vascular lesions. BRBNS is characterized by venous malformations usually present either at birth or within the first few years of life. Found predominantly on the upper limbs, face, and trunk, three distinct types of lesions may be seen. Type I lesions are large venous malformations that may increase in size, become disfiguring, and even obstruct vital tissues and structures. Type II lesions are the most common lesions encountered in BRBNS. Often nipplelike, they are dark blue to black, thin-walled, blood-filled sacks that are easily compressed and slowly refill (**Fig. 15A**). Patients may complain of pain or increased sweating associated with these lesions. Type III lesions are irregular blue to black macules that do not blanch with pressure (see

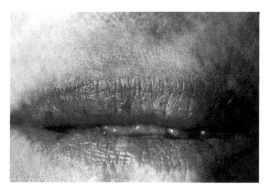

Fig. 14. Mat telangiectasias on the lips of a patient with hereditary hemorrhagic telangiectasia. (*Courtesy of* Marshfield Clinic Department, Marshfield, WI.)

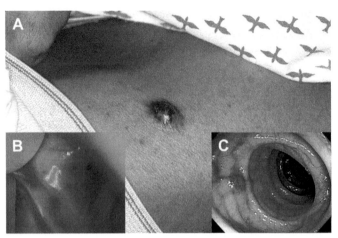

Fig. 15. (*A*) Nipplelike blue-black lesion of BRBNS. (*B*) Dark blue-black macules on the buccal mucosa. (*C*) Venous malformation seen on colonoscopy. (*Courtesy of* E.J. Stratman, MD, Marshfield, WI.)

Fig. 15B). These usually do not bleed spontaneously, become malignant, or regress; however, over time they commonly increase in size and number.[59,60]

The visceral manifestations of BRBNS consist of these same venous malformations, occurring most commonly in the gastrointestinal tract, predominantly within the small intestine (see **Fig. 15**C). They can lead to occult blood loss, intussusception, infarction, hemorrhage, or abdominal pain. Lesions in the eyes, thyroid, kidney, heart, lungs, adrenal glands, spleen, central nervous system, genitourinary system, and muscle have also been reported.[59] Diagnosis is made based on characteristic cutaneous findings. Histopathology can aid in this process. The lesions of BRBNS are true venous malformations and not hemangiomas. Most cases arise spontaneously, but there have been reports of cases of autosomal dominant transmission.[59]

POSTOPERATIVE DERMATOLOGIC CONDITIONS

Dermatologic issues often arise in the surgical patient during the postoperative recovery period. Postoperative wound infections can be dermatologic, but are beyond the scope of this article. During the preoperative and immediate postoperative period, surgical patients commonly receive many new medications. The first signs of adverse drug reactions to these medications or combinations of medications often involve the skin. By far the most common of these is the morbilliform exanthem. In addition, several chemicals in direct contact with the surgical patient's skin can lead to allergic contact dermatitis starting 1 to 4 days following the procedure. Rarely, surgical procedures can trigger a systemic dermatologic condition. Examples of such conditions associated with bowel bypass surgery and short gut are discussed.

Morbilliform Exanthem

There are more than 100 varieties of cutaneous adverse drug reactions.[60] The most common type of drug eruption is the morbilliform exanthem.[61] This eruption typically begins 4 to 14 days after beginning the offending medication, and rarely occurs during the first 1 to 2 days of use. The morbilliform exanthem consists of blanching erythematous macules and papules often beginning on the trunk with eventual spread to the extremities, head, and neck. In each region affected, the eruption typically expands from discrete lesions to eventual confluent erythema (**Fig. 16**). Many drugs given to surgical patients have the potential to trigger such a reaction, but none more commonly prescribed than antibiotics. The pathophysiology is complex and incompletely understood. Skin biopsy findings are not pathognomonic, and diagnostic tests are not readily available to determine which drug among many is the offending agent. The drug reference literature must often be used to determine the relative likelihood of one drug being the offending agent versus another, by comparing reported adverse reaction rates for the specific reaction type. Unfortunately, many drug reference manuals refer to many different types of cutaneous reactions as "rash," which is a nonspecific term. The two most helpful factors in determining likelihood of causality are time since medication onset and frequency of similar reactions reported in the medication literature.

Once the cutaneous drug reaction is identified, proper measures and expectations are important to avoid unnecessary cost, confusion, and delay to improvement. First, the suspected offending drug should be stopped if not essential or if adequate alternative therapy exists. Any nonessential drug should be discontinued as soon as possible, as many drug reactions are not caused by a single drug but by the complexities introduced by combinations of drugs, current infections, and other biologic factors. If there is no alternative to a critical medication suspected of causing the eruption, the medication can often be continued and the patient treated symptomatically. Management may include a topical steroid (typically triamcinolone 0.1% cream or ointment) soak and smear regimen.[62] However, the skin can herald systemic hypersensitivities affecting other organs. If continuing the suspected medication, fever curves, renal function, hepatic function, and joint symptoms must be monitored closely.

After stopping the suspected medication, the exanthem is unlikely to fade instantly. In many cases, the eruption will continue to expand in the 1 to 3 days following discontinuation, often progressing further down the extremities or becoming more confluent. This expansion is presumably due to further immunologic reactions with existing drug-related haptens already located in the skin at the time of discontinuation. After stopping the correct medication(s), most exanthems fade within 2 weeks. Eruptions continuing beyond 2 weeks postdiscontinuation should be reassessed for alternative drugs causing the exanthem. In most cases, morbilliform exanthems are pruritic, not painful. Painful exanthems should be evaluated for evolving toxic epidermal necrolysis, a more serious drug reaction with high morbidity and mortality. Topical steroid treatment with mid- to high-potency steroids are the best choice for

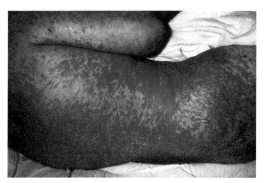

Fig. 16. Morbilliform exanthem with areas of confluent erythema on the lower back and right flank. (*Courtesy of* E.J. Stratman, MD, Marshfield, WI.)

safe, symptomatic relief. As the morbilliform exanthem is not a histamine-mediated process, antihistamine therapy alone is inadequate in most cases. The benefit of antihistamine therapy is related to sedative effects rather than direct influence on the skin eruption.

Allergic Contact Dermatitis

Many surgical preps, instrumentations, wound-care products, and dressing materials are known to cause allergic contact dermatitis in the postoperative period (**Table 1**).[63–66] Clinically, because of the intense erythema that can occur and the close proximity to the surgical wound, contact dermatitis can be confused with wound infection, particularly erysipelas. There are some distinguishing features. Whereas both conditions can be sharply marginated, contact dermatitis tends to be more geometric in configuration, is more likely to have yellow serous weeping, and is typically pruritic rather than tender, although some burning can be reported with contact dermatitis (**Fig. 17**). Biopsy can be helpful in distinguishing the neutrophilic infiltrate of erysipelas from the spongiotic, lymphoeosinophilic infiltrates of allergic contact dermatitis.[67,68] Mid-potency topical steroid creams may be selected for twice daily application, but should not be applied directly to the wound due to delayed wound-healing effects of topical steroids.[20,21]

Acrodermatitis Enteropathica (OMIM 201100)

Acrodermatitis enteropathica is a rare autosomal recessive disease due to defective zinc absorption in the duodenum and jejunum. Zinc is important for many physiologic processes, including metabolism of protein and carbohydrates, growth and development, wound healing, and cell proliferation.[69] It can be an acquired disease in patients undergoing bowel surgery resulting in short bowel syndrome, as well as celiac sprue, IBD, alcoholism, malnourishment, and vegetarianism. Clinically, pink scaly plaques

Table 1 Common surgical sources for allergic reactions	
Source	**Allergic Ingredient**
Topical antibiotics	Bacitracin
	Neomycin
Surgical metals	Nickel sulfate
	Cobalt chloride
Rubbers	Thiuram mix
	p-Phenylenediamine
	Carba mix
	Mercaptobenzothiazole
	Mercapto mix
	Black rubber mix
Anesthetic	Benzocaine
Disinfectant/preservative/ antiseptic	Formaldehyde
	Thimerosal
	Benzalkonium chloride
Adhesives	Colophony
	Epoxy resin
	Methylmethacrylate

Data from Jacob SE, Amado A, Cohen DE. Dermatologic surgical implications of allergic contact dermatitis. Dermatol Surg 2005;31(9 Pt 1):1116–23.

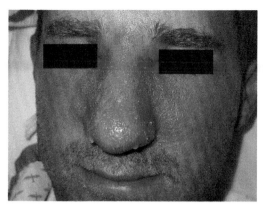

Fig. 17. Allergic contact dermatitis on the face following contact with dressing materials. (*Courtesy of* E.J. Stratman, MD, Marshfield, WI.)

resembling eczema are seen distributed around body orifices and distal extremities. The lesions may have a vesicular or bullous nature, and as the disease progresses, may take on a more erosive or psoriasiform character.[70] Other mucocutaneous manifestations include alopecia, blepharitis, angular cheilitis, paronychia, and stomatitis. Diarrhea, apathy, growth retardation, testicular atrophy, neuropsychiatric disturbance, and other signs and symptoms may be present. The classic triad of diarrhea, periorificial dermatitis, and alopecia is seen in about 20% of patients.[69]

If zinc deficiency is suspected on clinical grounds, a plasma zinc level is most commonly measured. This test should be performed after the patient has fasted, because meals decrease the zinc level, as does hypoalbuminemia. Inflammation may lead to increased zinc levels.[70] Once oral supplementation has begun, rapid clinical improvement is usually seen in 24 to 48 hours, even before increases in plasma levels. In cases of dietary deficiency, recurrence of lesions is seldom seen once sufficient oral supplementation has been achieved.[69] There is evidence that oral supplementation can also improve postsurgically acquired acrodermatitis enteropathica.[71]

Bowel Bypass-Associated Pustular Dermatosis

Bowel bypass-associated pustular dermatosis, also commonly known as bowel-associated dermatosis-arthritis syndrome, is a rare sterile pustular disorder that may have clinical overlap with pustular pyoderma gangrenosum and Sweet syndrome. Bowel bypass-associated pustular dermatosis syndrome, with its characteristic systemic and cutaneous symptoms, may be seen in up to 20% of patients who have undergone jejunoileal bypass.[72] This disease, now reported in patients with a variety of gastrointestinal diseases, including IBD, and those who have had gastrointestinal surgery resulting in blind loops of bowel, is characterized by skin lesions, fever, chills, arthralgias, myalgias, and general malaise. Onset ranges from days to years after bowel symptoms or surgery.[72] Lesions routinely begin as small erythematous macules that evolve to papules, sterile pustules, and papulovesicles over 48 hours (**Fig. 18**A, B). Distribution favors the trunk and upper extremities. Lesions usually resolve after 1 to 4 weeks. Recurrence of symptoms may be infrequent or as often as every 1 to 6 weeks. Larger, indurated, erythematous plaques or nodules resembling erythema nodosum may also occur.[72,73]

Pathogenesis involves bacterial overgrowth in the gastrointestinal tract, often in the surgical blind loops, which results in increased quantities of peptidoglycans released

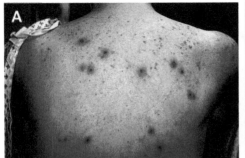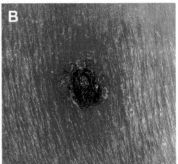

Fig. 18. (A) Lesions of bowel bypass-associated pustular dermatosis scattered on the posterior trunk. (B) Close-up of lesion showing a centrally crusted sterile pustule on an erythematous base. (*Courtesy of* E.J. Stratman, MD, Marshfield, WI.)

into the circulation. Immune complexes are then formed, and deposition of these complexes in the skin and synovium is believed to be responsible for the symptoms. Complement and antibodies to *Streptococcus* species, *Escherichia coli*, and *Bacteroides fragilis* have been identified in cryoprecipitates. Enhanced neutrophil chemotaxis and activation of the complement system alternative pathway may also play a role. Depending on the associated or underlying disease, patients with bowel bypass-associated pustular dermatosis have responded to antibiotics such as trimethoprim-sulfamethoxazole, minocycline, doxycycline, or tetracycline.[72,73] Other treatments include systemic steroids, treatment of IBD, or reversal of bypass. However, long-term treatment with systemic steroids is not recommended.[72]

SUMMARY

Preparation of the patient with preexisting skin disease for surgery can be challenging, and the medical literature is void of definitive, high-level evidence to guide decision-making and risk assessment. Nonetheless, by implementing treatment recommendations for commonly encountered skin diseases in cases when there are weeks between the initial consultation and the operative procedure, skin concerns may be lessened or even eliminated by the day of surgery. In addition, findings on the skin can assist the surgeon in identifying underlying causes for surgical complaints, presentations, or postoperative complications. In the case of genetic diseases, the surgeon can play a role in identifying situations in which an asymptomatic family member may also be at risk, thereby facilitating appropriate screening.

ACKNOWLEDGMENTS

The authors thank Marshfield Clinic Research Foundation for support through the assistance of Alice Stargardt in the preparation of this manuscript.

REFERENCES

1. Tzu J, Kerdel F. From conventional to cutting edge: the new era of biologics in treatment of psoriasis. Dermatol Ther 2008;21(2):131–41.
2. Weiss G, Shemer A, Trau H. The Kœbner phenomenon: review of the literature. J Eur Acad Dermatol Venereol 2002;16(3):241–8.

3. Saini R, Shupack JL. Psoriasis: to cut or not to cut, what say you? Dermatol Surg 2003;29(7):735–40.
4. Cheleuitte E, Fleischli J, Tisa L, et al. Psoriasis and elective foot surgery. J Foot Ankle Surg 1996;35(4):297–302.
5. Marples RR, Heaton CL, Kligman AM. *Staphylococcus aureus* in psoriasis. Arch Dermatol 1973;107(4):568–70.
6. Lynfield YL. Psoriasis in the operating theatre. BMJ 1972;4(5832):62.
7. Lambert JR, Wright V. Surgery in patients with psoriasis and arthritis. Rheumatol Rehabil 1979;18(1):35–7.
8. Stern SH, Insall JN, Windsor RE, et al. Total knee arthroplasty in patients with psoriasis. Clin Orthop Relat Res 1989;248:108–10.
9. Treadwell PA. Eczema and infection. Pediatr Infect Dis J 2008;27(6):551–2.
10. Williams JV, Vowels B, Honig P, et al. *Staphylococcus aureus* isolation from the lesions, the hands, and anterior nares of patients with atopic dermatitis. J Emerg Med 1999;17(1):207–11.
11. Brook I. Secondary bacterial infections complicating skin lesions. J Med Microbiol 2002;51(10):808–12.
12. Lin YT, Wang CT, Chiang BL. Role of bacterial pathogens in atopic dermatitis. Clin Rev Allergy Immunol 2007;33(3):167–77.
13. Beckett KS, Gault DT. Operating in an eczematous surgical field: don't be rash, delay surgery to avoid infective complications. J Plast Reconstr Aesthet Surg 2006;59(12):1446–9.
14. Hung SH, Lin YT, Chu CY, et al. Staphylococcus colonization in atopic dermatitis treated with fluticasone or tacrolimus with or without antibiotics. Ann Allergy Asthma Immunol 2007;98(1):51–6.
15. Janniger CK, Schwartz RA, Szepietowski JC, et al. Intertigo and common secondary skin infections. Am Fam Physician 2005;72(5):833–8.
16. Bernard P. Management of common bacterial infections of the skin. Curr Opin Infect Dis 2008;21(2):122–8.
17. Kawana R, Kitamura T, Nakagomi O, et al. Inactivation of human viruses by povidone-iodine in comparison with other antiseptics. Dermatology 1997;195(Suppl 2):29–35.
18. Stratman E. Visceral zoster as the presenting feature of disseminated herpes zoster. J Am Acad Dermatol 2002;46(5):771–4.
19. de Lathouwer OG, de Fontaine S. Iterative wound dehiscence in augmentation mammaplasty as a systemic side effect of hidden topical corticotherapy. Plast Reconstr Surg 2006;117(6):2097–8.
20. Hengge UR, Ruzicka T, Schwartz RA, et al. Adverse effects of topical glucocorticosteroids. J Am Acad Dermatol 2006;54(1):1–15.
21. Busti AJ, Hooper JS, Amaya CJ, et al. Effects of perioperative antiinflammatory and immunomodulating therapy on surgical wound healing. Pharmacotherapy 2005;25(11):1566–91.
22. Langley RG, Luger TA, Cork MJ, et al. An update on the safety and tolerability of pimecrolimus cream 1%: evidence from clinical trials and post-marketing surveillance. Dermatology 2007;215(Suppl 1):27–44.
23. Rustin MH. The safety of tacrolimus ointment for the treatment of atopic dermatitis: a review. Br J Dermatol 2007;157(5):861–73.
24. Wahn U, Bos JD, Goodfield M, et al. Efficacy and safety of pimecrolimus cream in the long-term management of atopic dermatitis in children. Pediatrics 2002;110(1 Pt 1):1–8.
25. Arboleda B, Cruz NI. The effect of systemic isotretinoin on wound contraction in guinea pigs. Plast Reconstr Surg 1989;83(1):118–21.

26. Moy RL, Moy LS, Bennett RG, et al. Systemic isotretinoin: effects on dermal wound healing in a rabbit ear model in vivo. J Dermatol Surg Oncol 1990;16(12):1142–6.

27. Tan SR, Tope WD. Effect of acitretin on wound healing in organ transplant recipients. Dermatol Surg 2004;30(4 Pt 2):667–73.

28. Graves JE, Nunley K, Heffernan MP. Off-label uses of biologics in dermatology: rituximab, omalizumab, infliximab, etanercept, adalimumab, efalizumab, and alefacept (part 2 of 2). J Am Acad Dermatol 2007;56(1):e55–79.

29. Hernandez C, Emer J, Robinson JK. Perioperative management of medications for psoriasis and psoriatic arthritis: a review for the dermasurgeon. Dermatol Surg 2008;34(4):446–59.

30. Ephgrave K. Extra-intestinal manifestations of Crohn's disease. Surg Clin North Am 2007;87(3):673–80.

31. Veloso FT. Review article: skin complications associated with inflammatory bowel disease. Aliment Pharmacol Ther 2004;20(Suppl 4):50–3.

32. González-Guerra E, Angulo J, Vargas-Machuca I, et al. Cutaneous Crohn's disease causing deformity of the penis and scrotum. Acta Derm Venereol 2006;86(2):179–80.

33. Hart AL, Plamondon S, Kamm MA. Topical tacrolimus in the treatment of perianal Crohn's disease: exploratory randomized controlled trial. Inflamm Bowel Dis 2007;13(3):245–53.

34. Lan CC, Yu HS, Wu CS, et al. FK506 inhibits tumour necrosis factor-alpha secretion in human keratinocytes via regulation of nuclear factor-kappaB. Br J Dermatol 2005;153(4):725–32.

35. Requena L, Sanchez Yus E. Erythema nodosum. Semin Cutan Med Surg 2007; 26(2):114–25.

36. Field E, Allan RB. Review article: oral ulceration – aetiopathogenesis, clinical diagnosis and management in the gastrointestinal clinic. Aliment Pharmacol Ther 2003;18(10):949–62.

37. White C Jr, Howard A. Non-infectious granulomas. In: Bolognia JL, Jorizzo J, Rapini R, editors. Dermatology, vol. 2. 2nd edition. London: Mosby Elsevier Limited; 2008. p. 1433.

38. Crowson AN, Mihm MC Jr, Magro C. Pyoderma gangrenosum: a review. J Cutan Pathol 2003;30(2):97–107.

39. Brooklyn T, Dunnill G, Probert C. Diagnosis and treatment of pyoderma gangrenosum. BMJ 2006;333(7560):181–4.

40. Cohen P. Sweet's syndrome – a comprehensive review of an acute febrile neutrophilic dermatosis. Orphanet J Rare Dis 2007;2:34.

41. Gene tests Web site. Available at: http://www.genetests.org/. Accessed August 27, 2008.

42. Callen JP. Skin signs of internal malignancy. In: Callen JP, Jorizzo JL, Bolognia JL, et al, editors. Dermatological signs of internal disease. 3rd edition. Philadelphia: Saunders; 2003. p. 102–3.

43. Giardiello FM, Trimbath JD. Peutz-Jeghers syndrome and management recommendations. Clin Gastroenterol Hepatol 2006;4(4):408–15.

44. McGarrity TJ, Kulin HE, Zaino RJ. Peutz-Jeghers syndrome. Am J Gastroenterol 2000;95(3):596–604.

45. Galiatsatos P, Foulkes WD. Familial adenomatous polyposis. Am J Gastroenterol 2006;101(2):385–98.

46. Muir EG, Bell AJ, Barlow KA. Multiple primary carcinomata of the colon, duodenum, and larynx associated with kerato-acanthomata of the face. Br J Surg 1967;54(3):191–5.

47. Schwartz R, Torre D. The Muir-Torre syndrome: a 25-year retrospect. J Am Acad Dermatol 1995;33(1):90–104.
48. Ponti G, Ponz de Leon M. Muir-Torre syndrome. Lancet Oncol 2005;6(12):980–7.
49. Gustafson S, Zbuk KM, Scacheri C, et al. Cowden syndrome. Semin Oncol 2007; 34(5):428–34.
50. Uppal S, Mistry D, Coatesworth AP. Cowden disease: a review. Int J Clin Pract 2007;61(4):645–52.
51. Winship IM, Dudding TE. Lessons from the skin – cutaneous features of familial cancer. Lancet Oncol 2008;9(5):462–72.
52. Requena L, Gutiérrez J, Sánchez Yus E. Multiple sclerotic fibromas of the skin. A cutaneous marker of Cowden's disease. J Cutan Pathol 1992;19(4):346–51.
53. Vincent A, Farley M, Chan E, et al. Birt-Hogg-Dubé syndrome: a review of the literature and the differential diagnosis of firm facial papules. J Am Acad Dermatol 2003;49:698–705.
54. Schaffer JV, Gohara MA, McNiff JM, et al. Multiple facial angiofibromas: a cutaneous manifestation of Birt-Hogg-Dubé syndrome. J Am Acad Dermatol 2005; 53(2 Suppl 1):S108–11.
55. Welsch MJ, Krunic A, Medenica MM. Birt-Hogg-Dubé syndrome. Int J Dermatol 2005;44(8):668–73.
56. Begbie ME, Wallace GM, Shovlin CL. Hereditary haemorrhagic telangiectasia (Osler-Weber-Rendu syndrome): a view from the 21st century. Postgrad Med J 2003;79(927):18–24.
57. Bayrak-Toydemir P, Mao R, Lewin S, et al. Hereditary hemorrhagic telangiectasia: an overview of diagnosis and management in the molecular era for clinicians. Genet Med 2004;6(4):175–91.
58. Garzon MC, Huang JT, Enjolras O, et al. Vascular malformations. Part II: associated syndromes. J Am Acad Dermatol 2007;56(4):541–64.
59. Nahm WK, Moise S, Eichenfield LF, et al. Venous malformations in blue rubber bleb nevus syndrome: variable onset of presentation. J Am Acad Dermatol 2004;50(5 Suppl):S101–6.
60. Litt JZ. Litt's drug eruption reference manual including drug interactions. 14th edition. UK: Informa Healthcare; 2008. p. 647, viii.
61. Gutman AB, Kligman AM, Sciacca J, et al. Soak and smear: a standard technique revisited. Arch Dermatol 2005;141(12):1556–9.
62. Ertem D, Acar Y, Kotiloglu E, et al. Blue rubber bleb nevus syndrome. Pediatrics 2001;107(2):418–20.
63. Rietschel RL, Fowler JF, Fisher AA. Reactions to selected medications and medical care. In: Reitschel RL, Fowler JF, editors. Fisher's contact dermatitis. 5th edition. Philadelphia: Lippincott, Williams & Wilkins; 2001. p. 109–36.
64. Rietschel RL, Fowler JF, Fisher AA. Antiseptics and disinfectants. In: Reitschle RL, Fowler JF, editors. Fisher's contact dermatitis. 5th edition. Philadelphia: Lippincott, Williams & Wilkins; 2001. p. 149–202.
65. Rietschel RL, Fowler JF, Fisher AA. Contact dermatitis in health personnel. In: Reitschel RL, Fowler JF, editors. Fisher's contact dermatitis. 5th edition. Philadelphia: Lippincott, Williams & Wilkins; 2001. p. 451–65.
66. Jacob SE, Amado A, Cohen DE. Dermatologic surgical implications of allergic contact dermatitis. Dermatol Surg 2005;31(9 Pt 1):1116–23.
67. Rapini RP. Practical dermatopathology. Philadelphia: Elsevier Mosby; 2005. p. 48.
68. Rapini RP. Bacterial diseases. In: Practical dermatopathology. Philadelphia: Elsevier Mosby; 2005. p. 157.

69. Perafán-Riveros C, França LF, Alves AC, et al. Acrodermatitis enteropathica: case report and review of the literature. Pediatr Dermatol 2002;19(5):426–31.

70. Maverakis E, Fung MA, Lynch PJ, et al. Acrodermatitis enteropathica and an overview of zinc metabolism. J Am Acad Dermatol 2007;56(1):116–24.

71. Suchithra N, Sreejith P, Pappachan JM, et al. Acrodermatitis enteropathica-like skin eruption in a case of short bowel syndrome following jejuno-transverse colon anastomosis. Dermatol Online J 2007;13(3):20.

72. Dicken CH. Bowel-associated dermatosis-arthritis syndrome: bowel bypass syndrome without bowel bypass. J Am Acad Dermatol 1986;14(5 Pt 1):792–6.

73. Ely P. The bowel bypass syndrome: a response to bacterial peptidoglycans. J Am Acad Dermatol 1980;2(6):473–87.

Local Anesthetics: Uses and Toxicities

Alan Harmatz, MD, FACS, ASPS

KEYWORDS

- Local anesthetics • Toxicities • Dosages
- Epinephrine • Administration

Minor surgery is surgery performed on someone else...whenever it's you it's not so minor...

Plastic and Hand Surgical Associates is an academic private practice that performs between 3500 and 4500 surgical procedures each year. About 95% of patients give our practice the highest rating possible on our surveys.[1] I am convinced that one of the main factors in meeting or exceeding patient expectations in surgery is our practitioners' expert and liberal use of local anesthetics (LAs). Indeed, I would say that, other than an alcohol swab, LAs are the most frequently used medications in our practice.

Surgeons are asked to do more and larger procedures as outpatient procedures as the economics of medicine evolve. Indeed, we all carry out procedures on an outpatient basis that only a short time ago we would consider only on an inpatient basis. Further, procedures that had previously been performed under a general anesthetic are now being performed under local anesthesia.[2,3] A good working knowledge of LAs will better enable the surgeon to meet those demands and to do so in a way that will enhance the patient's safety, experience, and comfort. Although the focus of this issue of *Clinics* is minor surgery, any meaningful discussion of LAs has to go a little further than a 3-mL syringe and a small amount of lidocaine.

HISTORY

Erythroxyion coca, or the coca shrub, has been used by Andean natives for centuries. The stimulatory effect of chewing coca leaves was investigated in the mid nineteenth century, leading to the isolation of cocaine in 1860 by Albert Niemann. An enthusiastic Sigmund Freud investigated cocaine's effect on mood and behavior, only to see the harmful and addictive effects it had on its users. Carl Koller was the first to use the numbing properties of cocaine in 1884, employing it as the first LA in ophthalmic surgery. As the toxicities of cocaine became better known, a search for other less toxic LAs was undertaken. In 1892, Einhorn synthesized procaine and the modern era of

Plastic and Hand Surgical Associates, 244 Western Avenue, South Portland, ME 04106, USA
E-mail address: ashpls@yahoo.com

Surg Clin N Am 89 (2009) 587–598
doi:10.1016/j.suc.2009.03.008
0039-6109/09/$ – see front matter © 2009 Published by Elsevier Inc.

surgical.theclinics.com

LAs was born.[4,5] The most commonly used LAs in our practice are lidocaine, bupivacaine, and prilocaine.[6]

PHARMACOLOGY OF LOCAL ANESTHETICS

LAs are agents that reversibly block action potentials at the level of the sodium channels, thereby interrupting axonal conduction. LAs' actions are nonspecific: they work on any nerve with a functioning sodium channel. Knowledge of the structural components of LAs will aid in better understanding how these interesting compounds work and perhaps why, sometimes, they do not.

LAs are composed of a lipophilic/hydrophobic group (an aromatic ring) connected by an amide or ester intermediate chain to a hydrophilic or ionizable group (a secondary or tertiary amine). Those compounds with highly lipophilic/hydrophobic moieties are more potent, more long lasting, and more toxic. This appears to be related to the site of action on the nerve cell membrane.[4,5,7–9]

The sodium pore channel is a complex entity. Its anatomy and function are not reviewed here. Suffice it to say that there is a hydrophobic entity in the sodium channel pore that has a binding affinity for the lipophilic/hydrophobic group of the LA. Binding can only occur with the sodium gate or pore in an open or stimulated position; LAs need access to get to their binding site. Once there, the LA stabilizes the channel in its inactive state and the nerve cannot repolarize. Only a critical length of nerve need be affected to stop conduction. The channel eventually recovers but at a speed 10 to 10,000 times slower than normal. The stronger the bond between the hydrophobic groups, the longer the effect. The strength and duration of this bond affect the therapeutic window, making it smaller, and hence influence toxicity.[4,5]

Amide linkages are less prone to hydrolysis than ester linkages and therefore influence the duration of effect. The hydrophilic group influences the onset of effect.

Metabolism of LAs relates to their duration of effect and to their toxicity. The more free LA there is in plasma, the more toxic it is. Ester-linked LAs are generally much shorter acting. They are rapidly inactivated by plasma cholinesterase. Amide-linked LAs are metabolized in the liver by the cytochrome P450 enzyme system. More than 50% of amide-linked LAs are bound to Alpha1 acid glycoprotein (AAG), a substance found in the plasma. Fluctuation in the levels of this important compound greatly influence metabolism.[4,7]

pH plays a very important role in LA function. LAs are for the most part poorly soluble amines. LAs are found on the surgeon's shelf as slightly acidic hydrochloride water-soluble salts. When injected into normal tissue, there is rapid equilibration of the pH, allowing the unprotonated compound to diffuse across the cell membrane. The cationic form of the LA binds with the sodium pore: ionization must occur after passage through the membrane in order for the LA to take effect. The charged form of the LA will not diffuse through the membrane; therefore, anything that alters the pH of the local milieu will affect the LA's ability to get through the cell membrane. The most obvious offender in this regard is local infection; here the environment is acidic, the LA is charged, and it cannot pass through the cell membrane to exert its effect.[4,5,7]

Nerve fibers have differing susceptibilities to the effects of LAs. These differences are most likely due to differences in fiber diameter and meylination. The small-diameter unmeylenated fibers, such as type C pain fibers, are the most sensitive to LA-blocking effects. Heavily meylinated, thicker fibers such as type A motor fibers are less so. Any fiber that requires an action potential to function, however, can potentially be blocked by the effects of LAs (**Table 1**).[5,10]

Table 1 Relative size and susceptibility to block of types of nerve fibers					
Fiber Type	Function	Diameter (μm)	Myelination	Conduction Velocity (m/a)	Sensitivity to Block
Type A					
Alpha	Proprioception, motor	12–20	Heavy	70–120	+
Beta	Touch, pressure	5–12	Heavy	30–70	+ +
Gamma	Muscle spindles	3–6	Heavy	15–30	+ +
Delta	Pain, temperature	2–5	Heavy	12–30	+ + +
Type B	Preganglionic autonomic	< 3	Light	3–15	+ + + +
Type C					
Dorsal root	Pain	0.4–1.2	None	0.5–2.3	+ + + +
Sympathetic	Postgangtionic	0.3–1.3	None	0.7–2.3	+ + + +

Data from Hondeghem LM, Miller RD. Local anesthetics. In: Katzung BG, editor. Basic and Clinical Pharmacology, 3rd edition. East Norwalk, CT, Appleton & Lange, 1987.

Aside from these characteristics, the single most influential component of LAs in practical use is the addition of epinephrine (EPI).

LOCAL ANESTHETICS AND VASOCONSTRICTORS

Vasoconstrictors in conjunction with LAs have been used to treat patients almost from their inception. Confusion and controversy regarding the use of vasoconstrictors with LAs may stem from a lack of understanding of how these drugs work and how they work together.

Two main catecholamines have been used in LA formulations over the years: EPI and norepinepherine (NE). EPI is by far more widely used. NE has fallen out of favor for good reason. These two compounds differ in the effect they have on the adrenergic system and on the effectiveness and toxicities of the LAs themselves.

The main areas of activity for the catecholamines are the alpha and beta receptors found throughout the body. Beta1 receptors increase heart rate and contractility. Beta2 receptors cause vasodilatation in pulmonary and skeletal muscle vascular beds. Alpha receptors increase vasoconstriction in peripheral vascular beds. EPI has both Beta1 and Beta2 effects, whereas NE has mostly Beta1 effects. EPI has a four-fold greater alpha effect than that of NE. EPI tends to improve ventricular diastolic function. Mean arterial pressure (MAP) in patients injected with LA/EPI tends to remain stable. EPI alpha effects prolong the effects of LAs by delaying their uptake by the local vascular bed and diminishing potential toxicity as well by slowing the rate of rise of LA serum levels. Local blood loss is decreased. EPI has a serum half-life of less than 1 minute. It is rapidly metabolized by catechol-O-methyl transferase in blood, lung, liver, and elsewhere. Those injected with LA/NE have impaired ventricular diastolic function. Patients become hypertensive with an elevation of MAP because of a lack of Beta2 effect. A compensatory vagal reflex results in rebound bradycardia. NE has no local alpha benefit; therefore, EPI is the better choice.[4,11]

TOXICITIES OF LOCAL ANESTHETICS

In a 2003 study evaluating adverse events during oral and maxillofacial surgery in the state of Massachusetts, the most common adverse event associated with the use of

LAs was syncope, occurring in approximately 1 in 160 patients. Nonetheless, 17 of approximately 180,000 patients suffered a seizure, and 12 had some sort of cardiac side effect. These statistics are in line with what is known about LAs: the most common toxicities are neurologic and cardiac. Deaths have occurred from inappropriate use of LAs. A recent report details a death from LA overdose. I encourage all to read it.[12–14]

Neurologic toxicity is frequently manifested as agitation, restlessness, and tremor. These effects are presumably produced by LA depression of central cortical inhibitory pathways, leaving the excitatory pathways uninhibited. Seizures can follow. Higher levels of LAs can lead to central nervous system depression, respiratory failure, and death. In high concentrations, LAs can be injurious to nerve tissue itself, causing sensory and or motor impairment.

Cardiac toxicity results from a two-fold mechanism, direct to the cardiac muscle and from dysfunction of the autonomic ganglia. Myocardial contractility is greatly impaired due to the conduction-blocking effects of LAs. This effect can be used to great advantage, however, as many patients have been saved from malignant dysrythmia by the timely use of lidocaine. True ventricular dysrythmias from LA overdose are rare, with the exception of bupivacaine, which can cause ventricular tachycardia and fibrillation. Cardiac side effects are usually seen with very high serum concentrations and most often follow neurologic manifestations.[4,5,7,12–15]

TREATMENT OF LOCAL ANESTHETIC TOXICITIES

Drug treatment of LA toxicities has undergone an evolution over the past decade. The most important part of treating LA toxicity, however, is recognizing it. Remember, the first sign may be simple agitation. Inadvertent intravascular injection of LAs is the fastest way to elevate serum LA levels and precipitate a reaction. Under such circumstances, injection or infusion should be stopped immediately. Adding medications such as hyaluronidase may actually worsen the situation by further elevating plasma LA levels. Supportive measures, such as supplemental oxygen, positional change, oxygen saturation, and blood pressure monitoring, are all appropriate. Until recently, benzodiazepines were the drug of choice for the treatment of neurologic side effects. Diazepam 0.1 mg to 0.2 mg.kg can be given intravenous (IV), intramuscular (IM), or per rectum.

Twenty percent lipid emulsion has been shown to reverse the toxic effects of LAs, both neurologic and cardiac, quickly and effectively. Several cases have been documented in the literature reporting patients saved from bupivacaine toxicity by timely infusion of 1 mg to 2 mg/kg of 20% lipid emulsion. The mechanism of action is not clear; however, it has be postulated that the lipid acts as kind of a LA sink, scouring the blood for LA and binding it, quickly decreasing the serum level, perhaps mimicking AAG. Allergies to LAs are quite rare. Nonetheless, true IgE allergic reactions can occur. A thorough history should be taken, and, if a full-blown allergy is suspected, then the patient should be referred to an allergy/immunology specialist for evaluation. Ester-linked LAs are most often linked to true anaphylaxis. Sulfites used to stabilize vasoconstrictors and methylparaben, a bacteriostatic agent similar to an ester linkage found in some LA, can cause non–IgE-mediated allergic reactions.[4,8,13,16]

There have been reports of prilocaine causing methemoglobinemia. Hydrolysis of prilocaine initially leads to the formation of o-toluidine products that can bind to hemoglobin and cause methemoglobinemia.[8,13,17]

Most reactions not related to LA toxicity can be classified into psychosomatic responses and idiosyncratic reactions. Hyperventilation, tachycardia, or vagal episodes may well be due to anxiety. They are treated supportively. Idiosyncratic reactions can occur with the use of prilocaine as previously stated. Methemoglobinemia causes cyanosis and is treated with 100% oxygen and IV methylene blue (which acts as an electron receptor and reduces the formation of methemoglobin). Newborns, patients with hemoglobinopathies, and those with glucose-6-phosphate dehydrogenase deficiency are at greatest risk.[13,16]

DOSING AND ADMINISTRATION TECHNIQUE

Dosing guidelines for LAs are vague. In fact, the recommended doses for the same LAs differ from country to country. Manufactures have issued dosing guidelines for LAs that are more empirically based rather than evidence based. The reason for this may be the companies' attempt to ensure a very generous margin of safety for these widely used medications; some of it may be out of liability concerns. To be fair, dosing of LAs is not straightforward. Comorbidities, anatomic location, and surface area to be treated as well as concentration of the LA, the addition of EPI, and rapidity of the infusion all factor into safe dosing guidelines (**Table 2**).[7,10–12,18,19]

PATIENT FACTORS IN DOSING

Much of what is contained within this section is in greater part derived from an excellent article by Rosenberg and colleagues.[7] The authors take a critical look at all of the factors involved in LA dosing.

Before injecting patients with an LA, it is important to consider their age, comorbidities, and medications, as all of these are factors in dosing decisions. Some of the recommendations that are noted below do not have any direct relevance in the minor procedure in the office setting. Nonetheless, they are important to mention as an aid in understanding these medications, thereby conveying informed caution.

The extremes of age are for the most part the most important factor to consider. Infants younger than 4 months of age have been shown to have higher plasma concentrations of LAs when given the adult equivalent dose. The reason postulated for this is the lower concentration of AAG found in plasma. Lower AAG puts this age group at risk for toxic effects at lower doses. Further, infants younger than 4 months of age appear to be more sensitive to bupivacaine. As a result, recommendation for lowering the dose of LAs by 15% is given to infants, especially those undergoing regional anesthetics.

The elderly, those older than 70 years, also deserve special dosing considerations. Diminished blood flow to those organs responsible for metabolism of LAs leads to decreased plasma clearance of LAs in those affected. Loss of fatty tissue and diminution in axonal function mean that the elderly are more sensitive to blockade of nerve function. Although there has been a report of an elderly patient who suffered the effects of LA toxicity at a lower serum concentration than had previously been reported,[13] plasma concentrations of LAs are similar to those found in younger age groups. The recommendation is for decreasing LA dose by 20% in those patients older than 70 years.

Renal impairment patients deserve special consideration. Lidocaine and bupivacaine have very different profiles in the patients.

Lidocaine appears to be very well tolerated. Lidocaine is metabolized by a hepatic route.[5] Plasma clearance of lidocaine is unchanged in the renal patient. Dosing guidelines are unchanged.

Bupivacaine has a lower plasma clearance rate in the renal impaired. In hyperdynamic uremia patients, bupivacaine shows a rapid rise in plasma concentration. Fortunately, AAG levels appear to be higher in this population. Increased AAG may act as a kind of safety mechanism or buffer, ameliorating some of the effects of renal

Table 2
Officially recommended highest doses of LAs in various countries

	Finland	Germany	Japan	Sweden	United States
2-Chloroprocaine	—	—	—	—	800 mg
With epinephrine	—	—	1000 mg	—	1000 mg
Procaine	—	500 mg	600 mg (epidural)	—	500 mg
With epinephrine	—	600 mg	—	—	—
Articaine	7 mg/kg	4 mg/kg	—	—	—
With epinephrine	7 mg/kg	4 mg/kg	—	—	—
Bupivacaine	175 mg (200 mgª) (400 mg/24 h)	150 mg	100 mg (epidural)	150 mg	175 mg
With epinephrine	175 mg	150 mg	—	150 mg	225 mg
Levobupivacaine	150 mg (400 mg/24 h)	150 mg	—	150 mg	150 mg
With epinephrine	—	—	—	—	—
Lidocaine	200 mg	200 mg	200 mg	200 mg	300 mg
With epinephrine	500 mg	500 mg	—	500 mg	500 mg
Mepivacaine	—	300 mg	400 mg (epidural)	350 mg	400 mg
With epinephrine	—	500 mg	—	350 mg	550 mg
Prilocaine	400 mg	—	—	400 mg	—
With epinephrine	600 mg	—	—	600 mg	—
Ropivacaine	225 mg (300 mgª) (800 mg/24 h)	No mention	200 mg (epidural) 300 mg (infiltr)	225 mg	225 mg (300 mgª)
With epinephrine	225 mg	No mention	—	225 mg	225 mg (300 mgª)

ª For brachial plexus block in adults.
Data from Rosenberg PH, Veering BT, Urmey WF. Maximum recommended doses of local anesthetics: a multifactorial concept. Reg Anesth Pain Med 2004;29:564–75.

impairment on bupivacaine metabolism. A decrease of 10 to 20% in those patients getting larger doses (regional blocks, continuous infusions via pump) of bupivacaine is recommended.

Hepatic dysfunction is an important consideration. Hepatic insufficiency rarely occurs alone. Other organ systems, renal, pulmonary, and so forth, are frequently involved, making dosing decisions in these patients even more complex. Amide LAs are mainly metabolized via the liver, so it would seem that hepatic dysfunction would greatly alter plasma concentrations of LAs. As expected, patients with end-stage liver disease have a 60% decrease in plasma clearance rates of LAs. Interestingly, those with mild impairment (alcoholics) have little change in their clearance rates. AAG may again play a role here, but it has been poorly studied. It does appear that even in end-stage liver disease, AAG continues to be made. Great care and due consideration need to be given to theses patients when administering amide LAs. Although up to a 50% reduction in dosing of LAs has been recommended for higher-dose repeat regional blocks, under normal office minor procedure circumstances, no reduction in dosing is recommended for isolated mild hepatic impairment.

Cardiac disease needs to be considered. A spectrum of patients from those with mild hypertension to those with significant heart failure needs to be treated differently. This relates to the degree of impairment of blood flow to lung, liver, and kidneys and its effect on plasma clearance of LAs. For patients with well-controlled disease, no dosage adjustment is required. For patients with more severe disease, a reduction of as much as 20% for repeat regional block has been recommended.[7,11]

The bigger concern for practioners with regard to use of LAs in patients with cardiac disease most likely has nothing to do with the LA itself, but rather the EPI is frequently the greater cause for concern. The best data on the outpatient experience comes from the maxillofacial literature, "Epinephrine and Local Anesthesia revisited" by Brown and Rhodus[11] All are encouraged to read it.

In short, EPI given to patients with well-controlled cardiac disease in conjunction with LAs in the office setting is safe and requires little in the way of dose modification. Addition of EPI to LAs slows their uptake and helps to diminish their potential for toxicity, a huge benefit. As previously noted, the Massachusetts study showed that 12 of 180,000 patients had some sort of cardiac side effect. I would postulate that at least a portion of those patients have side effects from endogenous NE released in response to pain from inadequate LA effect, an important fact to remember when trying to evaluate a hypertensive person in the minor surgery room.

A thorough review of a patient's medication should be undertaken before injecting any LA. Several medications influence the metabolism of LAs.

Amide LAs are metabolized by the cytochrome P450 enzyme system. Anything that inhibits a portion of that system impairs LA metabolism. In addition, some of these medications impair hepatic blood flow, further slowing LA clearance. Bupivacaine appears to be more greatly affected by these drugs than lidocaine. Propranolol and cimetidine are two such drugs and can impair bupivacaine clearance by up to 35%. The antifungal Itraconazole also affects the metabolism of bupivacaine similarly. Significant dose reduction in patients receiving repeat blocks is recommended.[7,16]

Epinephrine itself has been implicated as interacting with antidepressant drugs such as tricyclic antidepressants, monoamine oxidase inhibitors, and selective serotonin reuptake inhibitors causing hypertension. Change in beta-adrenergic receptors, specifically downregulation, has been postulated as the mechanism of interaction. A review of relevant literature does not support this conclusion; no case report has been published describing a link between LAs with EPI and TCA antidepressants. In the minor procedure office setting, LAs with EPI can be safely used in these patients.[16]

AAG levels are also affected by a variety of factors. Trauma, smoking, uremia, and surgery increase AAG levels in plasma. Oral contraceptives decrease levels.[4]

TUMESCENT SOLUTION AND LOCAL ANESTHETIC DOSING

LAs commonly used in the United States are 1% and 2% lidocaine with EPI 1:100,000 or 1:200,000 and bupivacaine 0.25% and 0.5% with similar EPI dilutions. Clinicians have modified these medications postmanufacture by mixing them, diluting them, and by adding bicarbonate to achieve their own particular cocktail. Plastic surgeons have taken this idea and created highly dilute solutions of LAs, EPI, and buffer. They are called tumescent solutions. A brief discussion of tumescent solutions will aid in further understanding the dynamic of dosing and toxicity.

Shortly after the first published reports of suction lipectomy by Illouz in 1977, surgeons began to look for ways to minimize blood loss, ease and enhance removal of fatty tissue, and improve patient comfort. First, a "wet" technique of infusing a large volume of fluid containing dilute hyaluronidase was used. To this were added low-dose EPI and dilute LA. In 1987, Klein coined the phrase "tumescent technique" and so it has been ever since. Though formulations of tumescent solution vary, a typical mixture would contain 0.1% lidocaine, sodium bicarbonate 12mEq/L, and EPI 1:1,000,000. The solution is usually warmed to approximately 37°C.[15,18,20,21]

As previously noted, the recommended dose of lidocaine in an otherwise healthy adult has been set at 7 mg/kg. Using tumescent solution, doses as high as 50 mg/kg have been administered without toxicity (although 35 mg/kg or lower is considered a safer dose); how can this be?[14,15,18] Suppositions that most of the LA has been suctioned out have not been validated. The explanation lies in the solution itself and where it is injected. Tumescent solution is injected into the subcutaneous space. When compared with plasma levels with IM or IV injections, subcutaneous levels are much lower. This is presumed to be due to the decreased vascularity of the compartment, leading to slower absorption. Diluting the LA and adding EPI with its powerful local alpha effects slows absorption even further. Add to these factors a relatively slow rate of injection and we go a long way in explaining why a 5-fold increase in the standard lidocaine dose is well tolerated.[7,8,11,19]

Not all areas of the body are created equal. In 2005 Rubin and colleagues[18] published an excellent study of plasma levels of lidocaine after infusion of a standard tumescent solution above the clavicles and then in the lower extremities. The plasma lidocaine concentration curves were similar in duration, meaning that by 14 hours postinfusion plasma levels of lidocaine were trending sharply downward. However, the average peak concentration from the neck infusion was 16% higher than that of the lower extremity. Further peak concentrations from the neck infusion were reached much earlier (5.8 hours) than those from the lower-extremity infusion (12.8 hours). Studies have shown that lidocaine toxicity occurs at approximately 4 mcg/mL. In studies using tumescent solutions with as much as 55 mg/kg of lidocaine, plasma levels never rose more than 3.6 mcg/ml.[14,15,18,22]

In summary, the risk of toxicity from LA use can be minimized by the following:

1) Using the lowest concentration of LA required; diluting is allowed.
2) Avoiding direct injection into the intravascular space.
3) Using EPI to slow absorption of LAs into the blood stream and to prolong anesthetic effect as well as minimize blood loss.
4) Modify the dose of LA/EPI for those patients with risk factors for toxicity.
5) Using enough LA to adequately anesthetize the area of interest.

TOPICAL LOCAL ANESTHETICS

Topical use of LAs has been employed since their discovery. More and more topical anesthetics are being used alone or in conjunction with injectable LAs. The absorption of topical anesthetics is related to the concentration of the LA employed, the amount of surface area covered, and the type of surface to which it has been applied. Systemic toxicity has been reported with the use of these compounds. A 22-year-old woman died in 2001 after application of 10% lidocaine/10% tetracaine cream from waist to feet for a laser hair removal procedure. Lidocaine applied to a mucosal surface can lead to plasma levels approaching that of parenteral administration. Care must be taken in the use of these compounds.[10,23,24]

Many surgeons are familiar with the combinations of topical compounds such as TAC and LET, which have been used in emergency departments for many years to anesthetize small lacerations. TAC is no longer in wide use as it has been largely replaced by LET, which has been shown to be just as efficacious, without the risks posed by combining cocaine and EPI (**Table 3**).

EMLA cream (AstraZeneca LP, Wilmington, Delaware) is currently in wide use. It is just one of a number of topical LA creams, but it is perhaps the best known. EMLA is a cream that contains 2.5% lidocaine and 2.5% prilocaine. It delivers maximal benefit after being in place for 30 to 60 minutes with an occlusive dressing. Systemic absorption of even large amounts of EMLA on large surface areas has been shown to be far below toxic levels. EMLA works very well in anesthetizing the skin before minor vascular access procedures and in superficial laser skin treatments. Though I was unable to find any report in the literature of methemoglobinemia from EMLA use, age-related guidelines have been issued to minimize the risk of this complication. EMLA is used on intact skin (**Table 4**).[10,25]

Special mention should be made with regard to compounding. Compounding pharmacies were until recently allowed to create or compound LA creams. High-dose creams, such as those involved in the death of the 22-year-old woman mentioned above, were made to order. The Food and Drug Administration put a stop to this practice in 2006 saying that these medications were not properly reviewed and that the pharmacies could no longer act like drug manufacturers.[26]

Table 3 Product descriptions				
Product	Composition	Time of Efficacy	Occlusion	Potential Side Effects
TAC	0.5% tetracaine, 1:2000 epinephrine, and 11.8% cocaine	30 min	No	Seizures: cardiac arrest
LET	0.5% tetracaine, 1:2000 epinephrine, and 4% lidocaine	15–30 min	No	None
Topicaine	4% lidocaine	30 min	No	Contact dermatitis
EMLA	2.5% lidocaine and 25% prilocaine	30 min to 2 h	Yes	Contact dermatitis; methemoglobinemia
LMX 4/5	4% or 5% liposomal lidocaine	15–40 min	No	None
BLT	20% benzocaine, 6% lidocaine, and 4% tetracaine	15–30 min	No	None

Data from Kaweski S. Topical anesthetic creams. Plast Reconstr Surg 2008;121:2161–5.

Table 4			
Guidelines for application of EMLA			
Age and Body Weight Requirement	Maximum Total Dose of EMLA (g)	Maximum Application Area (cm^2)	Maximum Application Time (h)
0–3 mo or <5 kg	1	10	1
3–12 mo and >5 kg	2	20	4
1–6 y and >10 kg	10	100	4
7–12 y and >20 kg	20	200	4

Data from Kaweski S. Topical anesthetic creams. Plast Reconstr Surg 2008;121:2161–5.

EPINEPHRINE IN DIGITS

I am often asked by students and practitioners alike if it is okay to inject EPI-containing LAs into various body parts, most often in the digits. The answer is yes, it is okay. When used to effect a digital block, EPI-containing LAs are quite safe and provide intraoperative hemostasis and postprocedure pain relief. As always, good judgment needs to be used: an insulin-dependent diabetic vasculopathic patient with a finger laceration might not be the best candidate for EPI injection in the finger.[27,28]

TECHNIQUE OF ADMINISTRATION

Delivering a good LA can be called an art form in and of itself. I have witnessed patients (other surgeons', not mine) writhing in pain, struggling to hold still while the surgeon, with beads of sweat collecting on his or her brow, attempts to deliver a small amount of LA. More often than not, this need not be the rule for administering LAs for minor procedures in the office setting.

A good LA begins with a good discussion. Make every effort to inform the patient of what to expect and tell the truth; telling the patient it will not hurt at all will only hurt your credibility with the patient. Every patient who elects to undergo a procedure under LA expects some discomfort. Be as specific as you can in telling the patient what will happen: where the surgery will take place, if they will need to change out of their clothes, what position they will be in, how long the procedure will take, and what monitoring precautions you may choose to employ. Tell them about the LA administration, how long it will last, and what to expect for discomfort. In cases of extreme anxiety, a topical LA can be placed approximately 1 hour before the procedure to alleviate the pinprick sensation of dermal penetration. If necessary, low-dose benzodiazepines can be prescribed to be taken 30 minutes before surgery.

The pain of injection of LAs is related to the site of injection, size of the needle, and the rapidity of the injection. The pH of the LA also plays a role in pain with injection. Injecting an area with a high concentration of sensory fibers, the tip of the nose, a fingertip, is much more painful than an area with lesser sensory representation, the thigh, the back. Small-caliber needles, 27 to 30 gauge, should be used to minimize the pain of dermal penetration. Inject slowly making sure that you avoid intravascular injection. This can occasionally be manifested by a sudden increase in pain as well as acute blanching in a vascular pattern. Adding a buffer to the LA has been said to decrease the pain of injection. Add sodium bicarbonate to the LA if desired. A 1 mL sodium bicarbonate to 9 mL LA ratio has been reported to work best. Do your best to be calm and reassuring but not patronizing.[29–31]

It has been said that dogs and children can smell fear. In our experience working with the latter, being calm and assertive is very important (this has also been said of working with the former). Maintain control of the room. Tell parent and child what will happen and do it. Do not wait for the child to give you permission; you may never get it. All you need is his or her understanding. Have everything you will need ready. Do not fumble around and draw up a 10-mL syringe of local with a 2-in long 18-gauge needle in front of a 9-year-old child and his or her mother. Try to transmit competence and inspire confidence.

Zilinsky and colleagues sum up all of these thoughts in a paper published in 2005 entitled, "Ten Commandments for Minimal Pain during Administration of Local Anesthetics." I encourage you to read it.[29]

The minor procedure room should have adequate lighting and a comfortable multiposition table capable of Trendelenberg positioning. Instruments, suture, and specimen containers should all be within arm's reach. Your preference for LAs should be present in abundance. Blood pressure monitoring equipment and an oxygen saturation monitor are essential. Supplemental oxygen should be readily accessible. Assistance should be close by.

SUMMARY

LAs are compounds unparalleled in their ability to alleviate pain. Surgeons with a good understanding of the actions and toxicities of these medications as well as the skill to deliver them will find that the minor procedure room is an enjoyable place for them and a comfortable and safe place for their patients.

REFERENCES

1. Patient Survey Review 2008. Quality Improvement Committee, Plastic and Hand Surgical Associates, South Portland Maine, quarterly report.
2. Carlson GW. Total mastectomy under local anesthesia: the tumescent technique. Breast J 2005;11:100–2.
3. Snyder SK, Roberson CR, Cummings CC, et al. Local anesthesia with monitored anesthesia care vs general anesthesia in thyroidectomy. Arch Surg 2006;141: 167–73.
4. Catterall WA, Mackie K. Local anesthetics. Goodman and Gillman's the pharmacologic basis of therapeutics. 11th edition. Chapter 14, Columbus, OH: McGraw Hill; 2006.
5. Hondeghem LM, Miller RD. Local Anesthetics. Basic and clinical pharmacology. 3rd edition. Chapter 24. Philadelphia; Elsevier.
6. Medical Supply Order Review 2008. Plastic and Hand Surgical Associates, South Portland Maine.
7. Rosenberg PH, Veering BT, Urmey WF. Maximum recommended doses of local anesthetics: a multifactorial concept. Reg Anesth Pain Med 2004;29:564–75.
8. Hunstad JP, Aitken ME. Liposuction and tumescent surgery. Clin Plast Surg 2006; 33:39–46.
9. Lindenblatt N, Beelussa L, Tiefenbach B, et al. Prilocaine plasma levels and methemablobinemia in patients undergoing liposuction Involving less than 2,000 ml. Aesthetic Plast Surg 2004;28:435–40.
10. Kaweski S. Topical anesthetic creams. Plast Reconstr Surg 2008;121:2161–5.
11. Brown RS, Rhodus NL. Epinephrine and local anesthesia revisited. Oral Surg Oral Med Oral Pathol Oral Radiol Endod 2005;100:401–8.

12. D'Eramo EM, Bookless SJ, Howard LB. Adverse events with outpatient anesthesia in Massachusetts. J Oral Maxillofac Surg 2003;61:793–800.
13. Litz RJ, Roessel T, Heller AR, et al. Reversal of central nervous system cardiac toxicity after local anesthetic intoxication by lipid emulsion injection. Anesth Analg 2008;106:1575–7.
14. Martinez MA, Ballesteros S, Segura LJ, et al. Reporting a fatality during tumescent liposuction. Forensic Sci Int 2008;78:e11–6.
15. Nordstrom H, Stange K. Plasma lidocaine levels and risks after liposuction with tumescent anaesthsia. Acta Anaesthesiol Scand 2005;49:1487–90.
16. Phillips JF, Yates AB, Deshazo RD. Approach to patients with suspected hypersensitivity to local anesthetics. Am J Med Sci 2007;334:190–6.
17. Clary B, Skaryak L, Tedder M, et al. Methehaglobinemia complicating topical anesthesia during bromchoscopic procedures. J Thorac Cardiovasc Surg 1997;114:293–5.
18. Rubin JP, Xie Z, Davidson C, et al. Rapid absorption of tumescent lidocaine above the clavicles: a prospective clinical study. Plast Reconstr Surg 2005;115:1744–51.
19. Ramon Y, Barak Y, Ullmann Y, et al. Pharmacokinetics of high-dose diluted lidocaine in local anesthesia for facelift procedures. Ther Drug Monit 2007;29:644–7.
20. Klein JA. Tumescent technique for liposuction surgery. Am J Cosmet Surg 1987; 4:263.
21. Sultan J. Effect of warming local anesthetic on pain of infiltration. Emerg Med J 2007;723–5.
22. Lillis PJ. Liposuction surgery under local anesthesia: limited blood loss and minimal lidocaine absorption. J Dermatol Surg Oncol 1988;14:1145–8.
23. Marra DE, Yip D, Fincher EF, et al. Systemic toxicity from topically applied lidocaine in conjunction with fractional photothermolysis. Arch Dermatol 2006;142:1024–6.
24. Shimron Y, Avery S. Woman had no lidocaine order. Available at: www.newsobserver.com. Accessed January 23, 2005.
25. Eldelman A, Weiss JM, Lau J, et al. Topical anesthetics for dermal instrumentation: a systematic review of randomized, controlled trials. Ann Emerg Med 2005;46:343–51.
26. The U.S. food and Drug Administration. FDA warns five firms to stop compounding topical anesthetic creams. Available at: www.fda.gov. Accessed December 5, 2006.
27. Thomson CJ, Lalonde DH, Denkler KA, et al. A critical look at evidence for and against elective epinephrine use in the finger. Plast Reconstr Surg 2007;119:260–6.
28. Waterbrook AL, Germann CA, Southall JC. Is epinephrine harmful when used with anesthetics for digital nerve blocks? Ann Emerg Med 2007;50:472–5.
29. Zilinsky I, Bar-Meir E, Zaslansky R, et al. Ten commandments for minimal pain during administration of local anesthetics. J Drugs Dermatol 2005;4:212–6.
30. Holmes HS. Options for painless local anesthesia. Postgrad Med 1991;89:71–2.
31. Randle HW. Reducing the pain of local anesthesia. Cutis 1994;53:167–70.

The Physiology of Wound Healing: Injury Through Maturation

Paige Teller, MD[a], Therese K. White, MD, FACS[b],*

KEYWORDS

- Wound healing • Skin physiology • Soft tissue injury
- Coagulation cascade • Fibroplasias

The physiology of wound healing is repeatedly described in medical literature. Most classic descriptions of wound healing consist of three phases: inflammation, proliferation, and maturation. However, the three phases of wound healing are not discrete events. The true complexity of healing evolves with increasing knowledge of cellular interactions and inflammatory mediators. The stages of wound healing occur both sequentially and simultaneously. Several variations exist in the recent literature, trying to create a framework for the molecular biology and cellular physiology of the healing process. The following description of wound healing provides a general summary of the events, cellular components, and influential mediators of wound healing over time.

INJURY

The initiation of healing starts with the creation of a wound. A wound is defined as an injury to the body that typically involves laceration or breaking of a membrane and damage to the underlying tissues.[1] Injury can occur from any number of mechanical or thermal forces that lead to disruption of the skin and damage to the connective tissue and vasculature. Bleeding ensues along with exposure of collagen, endothelium, and intravascular and extravascular proteins. This environment serves as a stimulus for hemostasis.

HEMOSTASIS

The resolution of injury begins with hemostasis. Vasoconstriction and clot formation lead to cessation of bleeding. Hemostasis is achieved through the activation of platelets and the coagulation cascade.

[a] Surgical Oncology, Emory University, 1365c Clifton Road North East, Atlanta, GA 30322, USA
[b] Plastic & Hand Surgical Associates, 244 Western Avenue, South Portland, ME 04106, USA
* Corresponding author. Plastic & Hand Surgical Associates, 244 Western Avenue, South Portland, Maine 04106.
E-mail address: twhite@plasticandhand.com (T.K. White).

Surg Clin N Am 89 (2009) 599–610
doi:10.1016/j.suc.2009.03.006
0039-6109/09/$ – see front matter © 2009 Published by Elsevier Inc.
surgical.theclinics.com

Vasoconstriction

Contraction of the smooth muscle within the endothelium is the first response to vessel injury. Reflexive vasoconstriction occurs before activation of platelets and coagulation. The endothelium of damaged vessels produces its own vasoconstrictor, endothelin. Other mediators for vasoconstriction are derived from circulating catecholamines (epinephrine), the sympathetic nervous system (norepinephrine), and the release of prostaglandins from injured cells.[2] Coagulation and platelet activation contribute additional stimuli for vasoconstriction through the following mediators: bradykinin, fibrinopeptides, serotonin, and thromboxane A2.

Coagulation Cascade

The coagulation cascade is made up of two converging pathways: extrinsic and intrinsic. The extrinsic coagulation pathway is an essential pathway for normal thrombus formation. It is initiated by exposed tissue factor on the subendothelial surface.[2] Tissue factor binds to factor VII and leads to the subsequent activation of factors IX and X. The intrinsic pathway is not essential to coagulation. As suggested by name, all components of the pathway are intrinsic to the circulating plasma.[3] Initiation of the intrinsic pathway is through the autoactivation of factor XII. Factor XII has the unique ability to change shape in the presence of negatively charged surfaces.[4] Factor XII, in its active form, is a stimulus for the activation of factors XI, IX, VIII, and X. Although each pathway has a distinct trigger, both lead to the activation of factor X and the production of thrombin. Thrombin serves two important roles in clot formation: a catalyst for the conversion of fibrinogen to fibrin and an initiator for platelet activation (**Fig. 1**).[5]

Platelets Adherence, Aggregation, and Degranulation

Platelets are the first cells to respond in wound healing. Activated platelets contribute to hemostasis through the process of adherence, aggregation, and degranulation. The presence of platelets at the site of injury is stimulated by exposed collagen and thrombin. Collagen within the subendothelial matrix comes in contact with blood flow, leading to the adhesion of circulating platelets. Platelet adherence is achieved

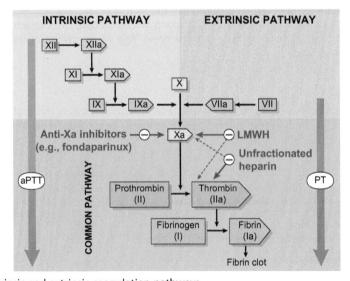

Fig. 1. Intrinsic and extrinsic coagulation pathways.

through interactions between platelet glycoproteins VI and collagen. Additional inter-actions occur between platelet glycoprotein Ib-V-IX complex and collagen-bound von Willebrand's factor. Platelet integrins play a supportive role in the adherence of plate-lets to collagen, von Willebrand's factor, fibrinogen, and other platelets.[5]

As mentioned above, tissue factor activates the extrinsic coagulation pathway leading to the production of thrombin. Thrombin is an independent initiator of platelet activation. Thrombin interacts with a receptor on the platelet surface (Par1) and leads to the release of ADP, serotonin, and thromboxane A2.[5] These substances enhance platelet aggrega-tion. Thromboxane A2 and serotonin also act as potent mediators of vasoconstriction.[3] Platelet aggregation in the environment of the fibrin matrix forms a clot.

Thrombus prevents ongoing bleeding, establishes a protective barrier, and provides a reservoir for substances released by platelet degranulation. Degranulation involves the release of numerous cytokines, growth factors, and matrix proteins stored within platelet alpha granules. These substances promote a variety of cellular and extracel-lular mechanisms important to hemostasis as well as several other stages of wound healing: matrix deposition, chemotaxis, cell proliferation, angiogenesis, and remodel-ing (**Table 1**).[3,6]

INFLAMMATION

Achievement of hemostasis leads to the immediate onset of inflammation. Inflamma-tion is evident through the physical signs of erythema, heat, edema, and pain. On a cellular level, inflammation represents vessel dilation, increased vascular perme-ability, and leukocyte recruitment to the site of injury. Two leukocyte populations sequentially dominate the inflammatory events of wound healing: neutrophils and macrophages. Both provide the critical function of wound debridement, whereas the latter also promotes ongoing cellular recruitment and activation necessary for subsequent steps in wound healing (**Fig. 2**).

Vasodilation and Increased Permeability

The establishment of vasoconstriction for hemostasis lasts only minutes before several factors stimulate the reverse response of vasodilation. Vasodilation is medi-ated by the presence of kinins, histamine, prostaglandins, and leukotrienes.[2] Vascular dilation increases blood flow to the wound, resulting in the characteristic inflammatory signs of erythema and heat. Increased flow also hastens the delivery of circulating cells and mediators to the site of injury. As vessels dilate, gaps form between the endothelial cells, increasing vascular permeability. Many of the same mediators of vasodilation (prostaglandins and histamine) also stimulate increased vascular perme-ability. Vasodilation in conjunction with increased permeability allows the transport of intravascular fluid, protein, and cellular components into the extravascular space. The extravasation fluid and migration of cells result in wound edema.

Leukocyte Migration and Chemotaxis

Although plasma passively leaks between endothelial gaps and proteins adhere to the wound matrix, leukocytes undergo the active process of diapedesis to enter the wound. Selectins provide weak adherence between leukocytes and the endothelium of capillaries. Stronger bonds are created between leukocytes, surface integrins, and intercellular adhesion molecules on the endothelial surface.[2] Cell migration from the endothelial surface into the extravascular space of the wound is mediated by numerous chemical factors and is known as chemotaxis. Chemotactic agents can include complement factors, histamine, bacterial products, prostaglandins,

Table 1
Platelet alpha granule components and their role in wound healing

Adhesion Glycoproteins	Proteoglycans	Hemostasis Factors & Cofactors	Cellular Mitogens	Protease Inhibitors	Miscellaneous
• Fibronectin	• PF4	• Fibrinogen	• PDGF	• α_2-Macroglobulin	• IgG, IgA, IgM
• Vitronectin	• βTG	• Factor V,VII,XI,XII	• TGF-β	• α_2-Antitrypsin	• Albumin
• Thrombospondin	• Serglycin	• Kininogens	• ECGF	• PDCI	• GPIa/multimerin
• vWF	• HRGP	• Protein S	• EGF	• α_2-Antiplasmin	
		• Plasminogen	• VEGF/VPF	• PAI1	
			• IGF	• TFPI	
			• Interleukin-β	• α_2-PI	
				• PIXI	
				• PN-2/APP	
				• C1 inhibitor	

Data from Rendu F, Brihard-Bohn B. The platelet release reaction: granules' constituents, secretion and functions. Platelets 2001;12:261–73.

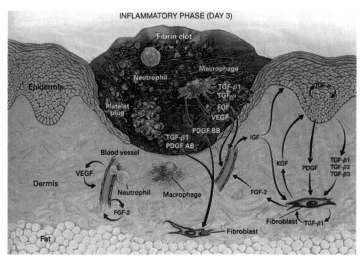

Fig. 2. Inflammatory phase day 3. (*From* Singer AJ, Clark RAF. Mechanisms of disease: Cutaneous wound healing. N Engl J Med 341:739, 1999; with permission. Copyright © 1999, Massachusetts Medical Society.)

leukotrienes, and growth factors. These substances recruit neutrophils, macrophages, and lymphocytes to the site of inflammation.

Neutrophils

Neutrophils are the first subset of leukocytes to enter the wound. Stimulated by prostaglandins, complement, IL-1, tumor necrosis factor alpha (TNF-α), transforming growth factor-beta TGF-β, PF4, and bacterial products, neutrophils arrive at the injury site in large numbers within 24 to 48 hours after wounding.[3–5] At this time point, neutrophils can make up 50% of all cells present within the wound. The primary functions of neutrophils are to defend the wound from bacteria and remove tissue debris. Neutrophils release several types of proteolytic enzymes, breaking down bacteria and extracellular matrix within the site of injury. Protease inhibitors protect tissue not involved in the inflammatory process. Degraded bacterial and matrix debris are removed from the wound by neutrophil phagocytosis. In addition to proteases, neutrophils produce reactive oxygen free radicals that combine with chlorine to make the wound less hospitable to bacteria.[7] The secondary role of neutrophils is to perpetuate the early phase of the inflammatory process through the excretion of cytokines.[3] One cytokine of particular importance is TNF-α. TNF-α amplifies neutrophil chemotaxis and stimulates macrophage, keratinocyte, and fibroblast expression of growth factors needed in angiogenesis and collagen synthesis. Neutrophils do not directly contribute to collagen deposition or wound strength.[3] In time, neutrophils are eliminated from the wound by either apoptosis or macrophage phagocytosis.

Macrophages

At 48 to 96 hours after wounding, the predominant leukocyte within a wound is the macrophage. Derived from extravasated monocytes, macrophages are essential to wound healing. They perform diverse tasks throughout both the inflammatory and proliferative phases of wound healing. Macrophages, like neutrophils, remove wound debris through the continuation of phagocytosis, proteases secretion, and bacterial sterilization. Serving as a primary source of numerous cytokines and growth factors, macrophages are necessary to support cellular recruitment and activation, matrix synthesis, angiogenesis, and remodeling. Unlike neutrophils, macrophages remain within a wound until healing is complete (**Table 2**).

T Lymphocytes

Attracted to the site of injury by interleukin-2 (IL-2) and other factors, T lymphocytes populate the wound to a lesser degree than macrophages. By week 2, lymphocytes represent the predominant leukocyte cell type within the wound. Lymphocytes are thought to be critical to the inflammatory and proliferative phases of repair. In addition to providing cellular immunity and antibody production, lymphocytes act as mediators within the wound environment through the secretion of lymphokines and direct cell-to-cell contact between lymphocytes and fibroblasts. The details of how lymphocytes contribute to healing are not fully understood.

Mast Cells

Another leukocyte recruited during inflammation is the mast cell. Mast cells can achieve a five-fold increase in number at the site of injury. Granules within the mast cells contain histamine, cytokine (TNF-α), prostaglandins, and protease. Degranulation leads to enhanced vascular permeability, cellular activation, collagen deposition, and remodeling (**Fig. 3**).

PROLIFERATION

The events of inflammation lead to wound debridement. Once debrided, wound healing enters a constructive phase of repair. This stage of wound healing is referred to as the proliferative phase. Proliferation takes place around postinjury days 4 through 12. During this time period, fibroblasts, smooth muscle cells, and endothelial cells infiltrate the wound as epithelial cells begin to cover the site of injury. In concert, these cells reestablish tissue continuity through matrix deposition, angiogenesis, and epithelialization.[3]

Fibroplasia and Myofibroblasts

Fibroblasts are one of the last cell populations to enter the wound. They are mobilized to the site of injury by products of the cell lines that came before them. The first signals for fibroblast recruitment comes from platelet-derived products: platelet-derived growth factor (PDGF), insulin-like growth factor (IGF-1), and TGF-β. The maintenance of fibroblasts within the wound is achieved through paracrine and autocrine signals. Macrophages and fibroblasts release numerous growth factors and cytokines that contribute to fibroblast migration: fibroblast growth factor (FGF), IGF-1, Vascular endothelial growth factor (VEGF), IL-1, IL-2, IL-8, PDGF, TGF-α, TGF-β, and TNF-α.[8,9] Of these substances, PDGF is the most potent chemotactic and mitogenic factor for fibroblasts and their progenitor smooth muscle cells.[3] Fibroblasts that migrate from surrounding tissue to the wound edge are activated by PDGF and endothelial growth factor (EGF) to proliferate and begin synthesizing collagen. Additionally, these fibroblasts are capable of producing matrix metalloproteinases (MMP). Secretion of MMPs allows for the degradation of the matrix obstructive to fibroblast migration.[2] There is a second population of fibroblasts that reside within the wound. Mediated by TGF-β, these "wound fibroblasts" differ from the fibroblasts that migrate from the surrounding tissue. They proliferate less, synthesize more collagen, and transform into myofibroblasts involved in matrix contraction. Fibroplasia is regulated by

Table 2
Macrophage activity and mediators in wound healing

Phagocytosis & Bacterial Stasis	Debridement	Cellular Recruitment & Activation	Matrix Synthesis	Angiogenesis
• Oxygen free radicals • Nitric Oxide	• Collagenase • Elastase • Matrix metalloproteinase	• Growth factors: PDGF, TGF-β, EGF, IGF • Cytokines: TNF-α, IL-1, IL-6 • Fibronectin	• Growth factors: PDGF, TGF-β, EGF • Cytokines: TNF-α, IL-1, IFN-γ • Enzymes: arginase, collagenase • Prostaglandins • Nitric oxide	• Growth factors: EGF, VEGF • Cytokines: TNF-α • Nitric oxide

Data from Diegelmann RF. Cellular and biochemical aspects of normal wound healing: an overview. The Journal of Urology 1997;157(1):298–302.

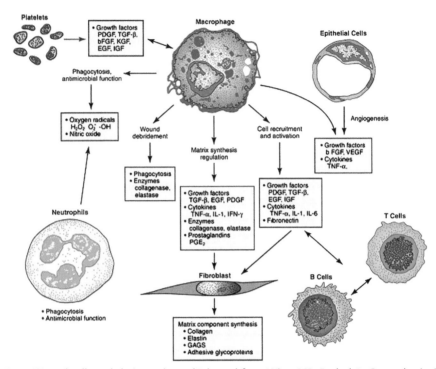

Fig. 3. Wound cells and their products: (*Adapted from* Witte MB, Barbul A. General principles of wound healing. Surg Clin North Am 1997;77:513.)

substances that inhibit fibroblast recruitment and mitogenesis: interferon-inducible protein (IP-10), interferons, and PF4.[10]

Matrix Deposition

In addition to mediating fibroplasia, PDGF and TGF-β play important roles in matrix deposition. Both of these growth factors stimulate the fibroblast production of a provisional matrix. The matrix consists of fibroblast-derived collagen monomer, proteoglycans, and fibronectin. Together these substances reestablish the continuity of connective tissue between the wound edges. As the matrix is created, TGF-β also functions to provide structural stability though decreasing protease activity, increasing tissue inhibitors of metalloproteinase, and augmenting production of cell adhesion proteins.[10,11]

Collagen and Proteoglycan Synthesis

Collagen, the most abundant protein in the body, exists in at least 20 subtypes.[12] Two subtypes are important to wound repair. Type I collagen predominates the extracellular matrix of intact skin. Type III collagen, present in lesser amounts in undamaged skin, becomes more principal in the process of wound healing. Collagen synthesis begins hours after wounding, but it does not become significant until roughly 1 week postinjury. The activation of fibroblast to synthesize collagen is derived from growth factors and the metabolic environment within the wound. Collagen gene expression is mediated by promoter-binding sites for corticoids, TGF-β, and retinoids. Increasing concentrations of lactate or the hypoxic environment within the wound can also stimulate collagen gene transcription and processing.[7] Lactate converts NAD+ to nicotinamide adenine dinucleotide (NADH). This depletes the availability of NAD+ to be converted into adenosine diPhosphate ribosome (ADPR). ADPR is an inhibitor of collagen mRNA transcription and other steps of collagen transport. Thus, a reduction in ADPR leads to increase in collagen mRNA synthesis. Collagen transcription occurs within the nucleus of the fibroblast. The transcribed mRNA is processed and translated by ribosomes. The resultant polypeptide chain has a repeated triplet pattern with a praline or lysine in the second position and a glycine in every third position. This protocollagen is roughly 1000 amino acids in size. On entering the endoplasmic reticulum, the protocollagen undergoes hydroxylation and glycosylation. The process of hydroxylation requires the presence of cofactors (oxygen and iron), cosubstrate (a-ketogultarate), and an electron donor (ascorbic acid).[3] Hydrogen bond formation is altered in the hydroxylated and glycosylated protocollagen chain, resulting in an a-helix. Protocollagen becomes procollagen as three a-helical chains wrap together in a right-handed superhelix. Procollagen is packaged within the Golgi apparatus and exported into the extracellular matrix. Within the extracellular space, a procollagen peptidase cleaves the ends of the chains, allowing for further cross-linking and polymerization. The covalent bond formation increases the strength of the resulting collagen monomer.[3]

In addition to collagen, fibroblasts produce and secrete glycosaminoglycans. Typically, glycosaminoglycans couple with protein to become sulfated, polysaccharide chains known as proteoglycans. Proteoglycans are thought to be a primary constituent of the "ground substance" of granulation tissue. As the collagen matrix replaces the fibrin clot, proteoglycans may provide a supportive role for the assembly of collagen fibrils.

Angiogenesis

Vascular damage incurred through wounding undergoes the restorative process of angiogenesis. Angiogenesis begins within the first 1 to 2 days after vessel disruption and can become visibly evident by approximately 4 days postinjury. Endothelial cells from intact venules migrate from the periphery to the edge of the wound. Replication follows migration and new capillary tubules form. Integrins (alpha$_v$, beta$_3$) upregulate on the endothelial cell surface, allowing for enhanced adhesion.[13–15] Proteolytic degradation of the surrounding wound matrix facilitates the advancement of new vessels across the wound.[13] In closed wounds, tubules from opposing edges quickly coalesce to revascularize the wound. Unlike closed wounds, the new capillary tubules of an unclosed wound merge with the adjacent vessel growing in the same direction, which contributes to the formation of granulation tissue.[7] The events of angiogenesis are regulated by a milieu of growth hormones (TNF-α, TGF-β, VEGF, FGF, PDGF) derived from platelets, macrophages, and damaged endothelial cells.[13] In addition to these mediators, the metabolic environment of the wound influences angiogenesis. Increased lactate along with decreased pH and oxygen tension contribute to a reduction in NAD+, an inhibitor of angiogenesis (**Fig. 4**).

Epithelialization

Much like angiogenesis, restoration of the epithelium begins early in healing, but it is not readily apparent until several days after wounding. Epithelialization reestablishes the external barrier that minimizes fluid losses and bacterial invasion. The process of epithelialization begins with epidermal thickening along wound edges.[3] Basal cells at the margins of the wound elongate.[2] Attachments between hemidesmosomes of the basal cells and the laminin of the basal lamina are broken down, allowing the cells to migrate. Migratory movements are facilitated by the expression of new integrins at the cell surface. Intracellular production and contraction of actinomycin also contribute to the forward progression of cells across the wound.[13] Epithelial cells

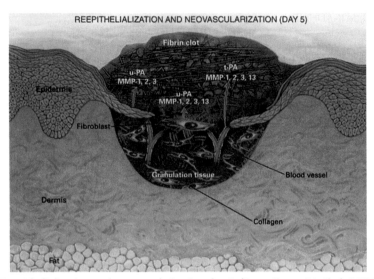

Fig. 4. Reepithelialization and neovascularization day 5. (*From* Singer AJ, Clark RAF. Mechanisms of disease: Cutaneous wound healing. N Engl J Med 341:739, 1999; with permission. Copyright © 1999, Massachusetts Medical Society.)

are capable of secreting MMP to breakdown fibrin in the course of their migration. The movement of basal cells parallels the direction of collagen fiber orientation within the wound, a process termed "contact guidance."[2] Epithelial cells will continue to migrate and proliferate until they come in contact with epithelial cells traveling from other directions. Contact inhibition signals the epithelial cells to cease their migratory effort.[2] A new monolayer of epithelium is created over the site of injury. Cells in this layer differentiate to take on a less elongated and more cuboidal or basal cell appearance. Hemidesmosomes bind once again to the basement membrane, reattaching these basal-like cells. Subsequent cellular proliferation leads to reestablishment of a multilayer epidermis.[2] The events of epithelialization are influenced by intercellular signals, growth factors, and the metabolic environment within the wound. Low oxygen tension within the wound leads to increased production of TGF-β. TGF-β helps keep epithelial cells from differentiating, allowing for ongoing migration and mitogenesis. TGF-α and keratinocyte growth factor (KGF) more directly stimulate cellular replication. Conversely, moisture and higher oxygen tension support the differentiation of epithelial cells to complete the later events of epithelialization.[7]

MATURATION AND REMODELING

In summary, the events of repair began with hemostasis and creation of a fibrin-fibronectin clot. Thrombus degradation followed with the arrival of inflammatory neutrophils and macrophages. Fibroplasia provided the ground substance made up of glycosaminoglycans, proteoglycans, and other proteins to support collagen deposition. New vessels navigated through this matrix as the new epithelium traversed the wound. The final events of repair remain collagen remodeling and strengthening.

Collagen Maturation

The last and longest event of wound healing is collagen maturation, starting 1 week postinjury and continuing for any where from 12 to 18 months. During this time period,

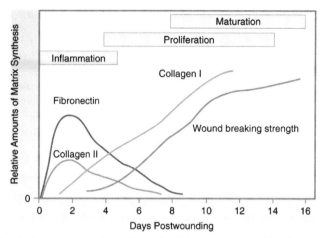

Fig. 5. Graph: relative amounts of matrix synthesis/Days postwound healing. (*Adapted from* Witte MB, Barbul A. General principles of wound healing. Surg Clin North Am 1997;77:513.)

the collagen matrix continually undergoes reabsorption and deposition to remodel and strengthen the wound. The initial collagen matrix differs in content and organization from that of uninjuried connective tissue. Intact tissue is composed of 80% to 90% type I collagen and 10% to 20% type III collagen. In contrast, the collagen matrix of an early wound consists of 30% type III collagen. The higher proportion of type III collagen contributes to a weaker matrix. Additionally, collagen fibrils within the matrix are more heavily glycosylated and thinner. These fibers are in a parallel orientation and do not interlace. At 1 week, the matrix strength is 3% of unwounded tissue. Collagenases and proteases cleave and degrade these early collagen fibrils.[11] This process is countered ongoing by collagen deposition. Newly deposited collagen increases in thickness, strength, and organization. Lysyl oxidase promotes cross-linking between fibrils.[11] With time, the ratio of type I to type II collagen approximates that of intact connective tissue.[7] By 3 weeks, the tissue strength increases to 30%. After 3 months, the tissue achieves a maximum of 80% its original strength (**Fig. 5**).[10]

Healed wounds are not capable of completely restoring the quality structure of intact tissue. The ability to closely approximate uninjured tissue is heavily dependent on size, depth, location and type of wound, as well as the nutritional status, wound care, and overall health of the patient.

An understanding of the basic science of wound healing is crucial to the clinician. Limitless intrinsic and extrinsic patient factors affect each step of this complex process. By understanding the underlying biology, we can significantly influence our patients' ability to heal.

REFERENCES

1. Merriam-Webster Dictionary. Available at: http://www.merriam-webster.com.
2. Lawrence WT. Wound healing biology and its application to wound management. In: O'Leary JP, Capota LR, editors. Physiologic basis of surgery. 2nd edition. Philadelphia: Lippincott Williams & Wilkins; 1996. p. 118–35.
3. Efron DE, Chandrakanth A, Park JE, et al. Wound healing. In: Brunicardi C, Andersen DK, Billiar TR, editors. Schwartz's principles of surgery. 8th edition. New York: McGraw-Hill; 2005.

4. Schmaier A. The elusive physiologic role of Factor XII. J Clin Invest 2008;118: 3006–9.
5. Furie B, Furie C. Mechanisms of thrombus formation. N Engl J Med 2008;359: 938–49.
6. Rozman P, Bolta Z. Use of platelet growth factors in treating wounds and soft-tissue injuries. Acta Dermatovenerol Alp Panonica Adriat 2007;16(4):156–65.
7. Hunt TK. Wound healing. In: Doherty GM, Way LW, editors. Current surgical diagnosis and treatment. 12th edition. New York: McGraw-Hill; 2006.
8. Eming SA, Krieg T, Davidson JM. Inflammation in wound repair: molecular and cellular mechanisms. J Invest Dermatol 2007;127:514–21.
9. Schugart RC, Friedman A, Zhao R, et al. Wound angiogenesis as a function of oxygen tension: a mathematical model. Proc Natl Acad Sci U S A 2008;105: 2628–33.
10. Broughton G, et al. The basic science of wound healing. Plast Reconstr Surg 2006;117(7S):12S–34S.
11. Diegelmann RF. Cellular and biochemical aspects of normal wound healing: an overview. J Urol 1997;157(1):298–302.
12. Adams CA, Biffi WL, Cioffi WG. Wounds, bites and stings. In: Feliciano DV, Mattox KL, Moore EE, editors. Trauma. 6th edition. New York: McGraw-Hill; 2008.
13. Martin P. Wound healing – aiming for perfect skin regeneration. Science 1997; 276:76–81.
14. Werner S, Grose R. Regulation of wound healing by growth factors and cytokines. Physiol Rev 2003;83:835–70.
15. Gillitzer R, Geobeler M. Chemokines in cutaneous wound healing. J Leukoc Biol 2001;69:513–21.

The Science of Wound Bed Preparation

Jaymie Panuncialman, MD[a], Vincent Falanga, MD, FACP[a,b],*

KEYWORDS

- Wound bed preparation • Debridement • Bacteria
- Moisture balance

THE SCIENCE OF WOUND BED PREPARATION

In recent years, advances in molecular techniques have led to increased understanding of the pathophysiologic problems encountered in chronic wounds (**Fig. 1**). The science of wound bed preparation (WBP) comes from technologic advances and their use in clinical practice. Technologic advances include new techniques in tissue culture, the development of recombinant growth factors, and tissue engineering. The identification of the components of the extracellular matrix (ECM) and how the balance of proteinases and their inhibitors affects chronic wound healing has been critical to our understanding.[1] The development of genetically engineered mice or mice models with knock-out features or the presence of inducible genes provided powerful clues to the actions of growth factors.[2] The cloning of growth factors and cytokines has opened the doors for gene therapy. Gene array technology is providing us with an understanding of the functional pathways and interactions of cellular components that carry out or regulate the healing process.[3] In essence, gene array technology allows us to identify the transcriptional profile of a large number of genes.[4–6] In the near future, this technology also might provide us with a powerful diagnostic tool to identify the specific processes that are impaired in a certain patient.[7]

The second area involving the science of WBP is how these new principles or treatments are translated into practice. These are discussed in detail.

ASSESSMENT OF THE PATIENT

To optimize the wound bed, the first step is to address systemic factors that are present in a patient and that impair healing. For example, one cannot expect healing

---

This article originally appeared in the October 2007 issue of *Clinics in Plastic Surgery*.

This study was funded by National Institutes of Health grants (DK067836 and P20RR018757) and the Wound Biotechnology Foundation.

a Department of Dermatology and Skin Surgery, Roger Williams Medical Center, Providence, RI, USA

b Department of Dermatology and Biochemistry, Boston University, Boston, MA, USA

* Corresponding address. Department of Dermatology, Roger Williams Medical Center, 50 Maude Street, Providence, RI 02908.

E-mail address: vfalanga@bu.edu (V. Falanga).

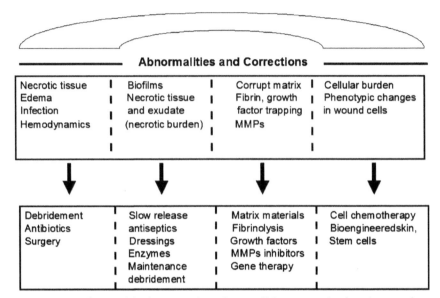

Abnormalities and Corrections

Necrotic tissue	Biofilms	Corrupt matrix	Cellular burden
Edema	Necrotic tissue	Fibrin, growth	Phenotypic changes
Infection	and exudate	factor trapping	in wound cells
Hemodynamics	(necrotic burden)	MMPs	

Debridement	Slow release	Matrix materials	Cell chemotherapy
Antibiotics	antiseptics	Fibrinolysis	Bioengineeredskin,
Surgery	Dressings	Growth factors	Stem cells
	Enzymes	MMPs inhibitors	
	Maintenance	Gene therapy	
	debridement		

Fig. 1. Overview of wound bed preparation, abnormalities present in chronic wounds, and possible corrective measures. Dashed lines represent the overlap among different compartments and corrective measures. (*Courtesy of* V. Falanga, MD, Boston, MA. Copyright © 2007.)

to take place without controlling edema in patients who have venous leg ulcers. The arterial component must be adequate as well. Tight glycemic control in patients who have diabetes is a priority. The use of off-loading footwear in neuropathic ulcers is imperative. Improving the patient's nutritional status also helps with healing. Evaluation for an inflammatory cause of nonhealing ulcers should be done if the ulcers are accompanied by signs or symptoms suggestive of a connective tissue disease. Finally, smoking cessation always should be part of the overall management.

NEED FOR DEBRIDEMENT

The first hurdle in applying the concepts of WBP is the confusion that proper WBP can be achieved solely by debridement. Debridement is definitely an important part of WBP; however, debridement alone is not enough to sustain healing in a chronic ulcer. An old, simplistic way of approaching chronic wounds is to think that one can transform the chronic wound into an acute wound by surgical debridement; however, this approach is not enough for the other underlying processes in chronic wounds. A better way of understanding the significance of debridement in chronic wounds is to think of debridement as a way to "introduce" an acute wound in a chronic wound.[8] Also, the chronic wound tends to accumulate a "necrotic burden" of senescent cells, a corrupt ECM, and inflammatory enzymes that need to be removed continuously without removing new, healthier tissues.[8]

When one is faced with necrotic eschars or gangrene in the context of life- or limb-threatening infections, surgical debridement is critical. Debridement also gives the clinician the advantage of accurately assessing the severity and extent of the wounds[9] Surgical debridement is the fastest way to debride a wound, but it is not selective because it removes viable tissue as well. "Maintenance debridement" in between surgical debridement interventions may be achieved by other methods, such as autolytic, chemical, or biologic means (**Fig. 2**).

Mechanical methods of debridement, such as wet to dry dressings, hydrotherapy, irrigation, and the use of dextranomers, is similar to sharp debridement. Mechanical debridement is fast, but nonselective and painful, and it generally is used for wounds with larger amounts of necrotic tissue.[9] In a study done to test the efficacy of growth factors in diabetic ulcers, ulcers treated with growth factors and debridement fared better than did those treated with growth factors alone.[10]

Autolytic debridement occurs by using the body's own endogenous proteolytic enzymes and phagocytic cells in clearing up necrotic debris. This process is facilitated by the use of moisture-retentive dressings[11] and may take weeks. Chemical debridement uses proteolytic enzymes to digest necrotic tissue. Enzymatic agents that degrade DNA or pancreatic enzymes that degrade proteins have been used in the past. Currently, two enzymatic preparations are in use in the United States: papain-urea and collagenase. For practical reasons, we focus on these two agents. Papain comes from the plant *Carica papaya*. Papain attacks and breaks down protein with cysteine residues.[8] Urea is added to this system to potentiate the action of papain by altering the tertiary structure of proteins, thus exposing the cysteine residues.[12] This enzyme preparation is active over a broad pH range (3.0–12) and is associated with an intense inflammatory response and breakdown of the viable portions of the wound bed. Use of these agents is associated with considerable pain.[8] Another formulation of this enzyme system was made with the addition of chlorophyllin. Chlorophyllin was added to address the issue of pain associated with papain-urea. Papain is not effective in debriding denatured collagen because the latter has no cysteine residues. In summary, papain is nonselective, but it has a broad spectrum of action and is useful in bulk debridement of relatively insensate areas.[8] The other enzyme used commonly is collagenase derived from *Clostridium histolyticum*. It is a water-based proteinase that specifically attacks and breaks down native collagen and acts in a restrictive pH range of 6 to 8. One advantage of collagenase is that it is extremely

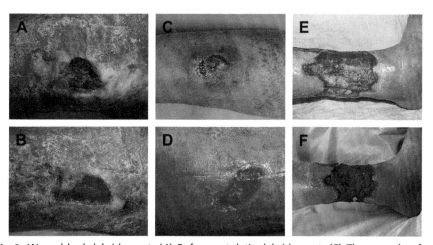

Fig. 2. Wound bed debridement. (*A*) Before autolytic debridement. (*B*) Three weeks after autolytic debridement. (*C*) Before surgical debridement. (*D*) One week after surgical debridement. (*E*) Before application of *Lucila serricata*. (*F*) Two days after application of *Lucila serricata*. (*Courtesy of* V. Falanga, MD, Boston, MA. Copyright © 2007.)

gentle on viable cells. Collagenase may be useful in the "maintenance phase" of wound debridement when one would like to break down tissue gradually.[8]

There has been recent interest in biosurgery, which involves the use of the larvae of the green bottlefly (*Lucila serricata*). This method has been used in patients with large ulcers having significant necrotic material that is not amenable to surgical debridement. The larvae digest the necrotic material and secrete enzymes that are bactericidal. Larva therapy is reported to be effective against methicillin-resistant *Staphylococcus aureus* (MRSA) and beta-hemolytic streptococcus.[13] Wounds are debrided in 2 days, debridement is selective, and side effects are limited to patient discomfort. This method of debridement may be done at home with the services of a trained nurse.[14]

The issue with debridement is to know when to stop. Traditional practice in acute wounds has been to debride to the level of bleeding tissue. In a recently published article, Falanga and colleagues[15] reviewed a method of wound bed scoring in which the presence of fibrinous slough did not affect healing adversely. In chronic wounds, because removal of the debris is part of a continuous process, debridement must be done without injuring viable tissue. It seems reasonable to state that the goal of debridement is to facilitate the efficacy of other treatments, be it growth factors, bioengineered skin, or topical antiseptics.

BACTERIAL BURDEN AND BIOFILMS

The role of bacteria in the healing or nonhealing of chronic wounds has always been a controversial topic. Although sterility of the chronic wound bed cannot be achieved, control of bacterial burden, in terms of bacterial density and pathogenicity, is a goal in WBP.[16] An important point in discussing bacterial burden in chronic wounds is the impact of host response. How one patient reacts to the bacterial burden is different from how the next patient reacts. Therefore, generalizations in handling bacterial burden should be made with caution. The presence of clinical infection is always a deterrent to wound healing. Clinical infection is the presence of multiplying bacteria in body tissues that results in spreading cellular injury as a result of toxins, competitive metabolism, and inflammation.[17] The cardinal features of an infection, such as heat, swelling, surrounding erythema, and pain, are still the standards by which infection is diagnosed; however, in chronic wounds, distinguishing a true infection from colonization often is difficult. It has been suggested that increasing ulcer size, increased exudate, and friable granulation tissue also are signs that should be considered in diagnosing an infection.[18] In light of increasing antibiotic resistance, we are faced with the challenge of antibiotic use. When then, does the presence of bacteria in the wound become a deterrent to healing? All chronic wounds are colonized with bacteria. Colonization is defined as the presence of replicating bacteria and adherent microorganisms without tissue damage.[19] Critical colonization is a recently defined concept that has yet to be characterized definitively.[20] This novel concept states that the bacterial burden in the chronic wound does not elicit the typical symptoms of an infection, but delays healing.[21] White and Cutting[22] proposed that this occurs because the bacteria in the wound do not incite an intense inflammatory response through the production of proteins that make them evade the immune system effectively; thus, the classic signs of infection are absent, but there is delayed healing through the inhibition of the growth of key cells in healing or by the presence of biofilms.[23] Biofilms are complex communities of bacteria that have evolved ways to communicate with each other through water channels and have a protective extracellular polysaccharide matrix covering. Through these communication channels, the bacterial colonies are able to up-regulate or down-regulate transcription of genes and protein products that are beneficial to them and detrimental to the host by a phenomenon called quorum sensing. Biofilms have high resistance to antibiotics.[24,25] Bacterial biofilms have been reported from isolates taken from chronic wounds;[26,27] however, more rigorous studies are needed.

The importance of the concept of critical colonization in the science of WBP is to encourage clinicians to pay closer attention to delayed healing and its assessment.[22] In instances in which healing does not take place, despite optimum treatment, critical colonization should be considered.[22] Obtaining and interpreting microbiologic diagnostic data always must be correlated with clinical findings. With regard to appropriate sampling methods, several studies established that properly done wound swabs were predictive of cultures grown from tissue biopsies.[28–36] The relevance of quantitative versus qualitative reports of microbiologic data in wound healing has been debated often. A critical bacterial load, synergistic relationship between microorganisms, and the presence of specific pathogens have been implicated in the development of infections and nonhealing.[37] Although studies were done in wounds of different etiologies, collectively the findings support the idea that the presence of 10^6 or more colony-forming units of bacteria per gram of tissue predicts delayed wound healing and a high risk for developing infections.[38–43] The detrimental effect of specific microorganisms on wound healing also has been studied. Most chronic wounds have a polymicrobial flora. It has been suggested that the presence in the wound bed of four or more organisms, rather than their type, is a predictor of nonhealing.[35,44,45] The reason for this finding is that certain microorganisms exhibit synergism. The importance of anaerobes in chronic wounds has been underestimated, possibly because of the difficulty in transporting and growing these bacteria.[21] The presence of beta-hemolytic streptococcus has been established to cause delayed wound healing or worsening of chronic ulcers.[37,44] The data on *Staphylococcus aureus* and *Pseudomonas aureginosa* as major contributors to delayed healing have not been consistent; however, other investigators showed that resident microorganisms have little effect on the outcome of healing.[46–50]

The indication for the use of topical antimicrobials is limited. The incidence of antimicrobial resistance is attributed, in part, to the use of topical antimicrobials that have a systemic counterpart. In addition, these topical antibiotics are potent sensitizers.[21,51–53] Mupirocin is effective in eradicating MRSA; however, because of its widespread use, the incidence of resistance also is increasing. Thus, interest in the use of topical antiseptics has been revived. Topical antiseptics have long been used but fell out of favor because of in vitro studies suggesting cellular toxicity; however, innovative formulations of antiseptics have allayed this fear. Cadexomer iodine and sustained-release silver dressings are examples. Topical antiseptics have a broad spectrum of bacterial coverage and deliver high concentrations of the drug to the wound bed; they also may be effective against biofilms.[17] In addition, silver dressings are useful in preventing cross-contamination of wounds and act as a barrier to the spread of MRSA, which is a useful feature in situations in which patients are in close contact with each other.[54] Debridement is an important adjunct in controlling the bacterial burden in wounds; it decreases the necrotic material and removes possible biofilms in the wounds.

In summary, surface swabbing may be an effective method for identifying and quantifying the bacteria present, but this needs further study. Wounds that are malodorous or exudative should be analyzed for the presence of anaerobic bacteria. Systemic antibiotics or topical antiseptics should only be prescribed in patients who are clinically infected or exhibit critical colonization. The routine use of antibiotics to facilitate wound healing is not supported by evidence. In the case of critical colonization, topical antiseptics may offer a first line of treatment. If a wound fails to improve after an initial course of 2 to 3 weeks, continued use is unlikely to be of any benefit. Systemic antibiotic therapy should then be considered.[21]

MOISTURE BALANCE AND DRESSINGS

A major advance in the way that we treat wounds has been the realization that moist wound healing is beneficial to nonhealing wounds and that occlusive dressings do not increase the risk for infection.[55,56] This discovery heralded the production of a variety of dressings that provide the wound with a moist healing environment and decrease pain, odor, and drainage. In chronic wounds, the wound fluid retards cellular proliferation and angiogenesis[57,58] and contains excessive levels of matrix metalloproteinases that break down matrix proteins, growth factors, and cytokines.[59–61] There are different types of dressings. An ideal dressing for chronic ulcers is one that provides a moist environment, absorbs exudate, prevents maceration of surrounding tissue, is impermeable to bacteria, does not cause allergies, does not cause reinjury upon removal, and is cost-effective. Unfortunately, no single dressing can accomplish all of these goals. The choice of dressing depends on the characteristics of the wound bed of a patient at a given time. Furthermore, a systematic review reported no therapeutic advantage to using different dressings for venous ulcers treated with compression, implying that dressings alone will not be able to heal chronic wounds.[62] Nevertheless, dressings are important because their use helps patients with their wound management and may prepare the wound bed for other therapies. We briefly discuss the types of dressings available.

Dressings that maintain a moist wound environment are described as being moisture retentive. This property is measured by the moisture vapor transmission rate (MVTR).[63,64] A dressing is moisture retentive when its MVTR is less than 840 g/m^2/24 hours.[65] The MVTR of hydrocolloids is less than 300 g/m^2/24 hours, in contrast to gauze, which has a moisture transmission rate of 1200 g/m^2/24 hours.[63] Depending on whether one wants to create a moist healing environment or if the control of heavy exudate is the primary goal, the MVTR is a useful tool in prescribing dressings. **Table 1** summarizes the properties of each dressing class and its indications.

An additional therapeutic advantage of dressings is the incorporation of topical antiseptics in their formulation. Topical antiseptics play a role in the control of the bacterial burden in the chronic wound. We focus on the newer topical antiseptics available: cadexomer iodine and silver. Both antiseptics are broad-spectrum antimicrobials. In addition, research has shown that they may be effective against biofilms;[66,67] however, in some studies, silver was cytotoxic in vitro to the host's own cells in a concentration-dependent manner. These in vitro findings do not necessarily translate to clinical practice. In addition, newer formulations of these antiseptics that are designed to release the drugs into the wound bed at continuous low concentrations helps to negate these cytotoxicity concerns. Striking a balance between controlling the bacterial burden and potentially harming dividing cells must be taken into consideration.

Iodine is a useful bacteriostatic and bactericidal agent that is effective against MRSA and other pathogens in vitro. The cadexomer is a polysaccharide starch lattice containing 0.9% elemental iodine released on exposure to exudates.[68] The antimicrobial activity of this dressing lasts for days, depending on its formulation. Cadexomer iodine is available in pads or as a gel. Upon absorption of water the lattice swells, releases iodine into the wound bed, and leads to a visible color change of the gel

Table 1
Summary of dressings and their characteristics

Dressing Type/Material	MVTR	Properties
Films (polyurethane film)	300–800	No absorptive capacity
Hydrocolloids (carboxymethyl cellulose, pectin, gelatin, guar gum)	<300	Not for infected wounds or heavily exudative wounds Traumatic removal High incidence of allergic contact dermatitis May produce offensive odor
Foams (polyurethane)	800–5000	For highly exuding wounds, not for dry wounds Used under compression bandages
Absorptive wound fillers (calcium alginate; starch copolymers)		Effective in undermined or tunneling wounds Nontraumatic removal High absorptive capacity Hemostatic properties Nontoxic and nonallergenic Improve pain May adhere to dry wounds
Hydrogels (water, polymers, humectants)		For wound hydration, not significant exudate absorption For minimally exuding wounds Not for use on a dry ischemic ulcer Nonadhesive Relieve pain May be used to moisten gauze packing
Gauze	1200	For heavily exuding wounds May adhere to viable areas of the wound bed Useful as a secondary dressing to contact layers

Data from Seaman S. Dressing selection in chronic wound management. J Am Podiatr Med Assoc 2002;92(1):24–33.

from dark brown to gray. Cadexomer iodine has been studied extensively and is safe and effective in reducing bioburden.[69]

Silver has been used for ages as an antiseptic from the formulation of silver nitrate to silver sulfadiazine. Silver has proven effective as an antiseptic with minimal toxicity. Silver is an element and is inert in its metallic form; however, once in contact with body fluid, it ionizes and becomes reactive.[70] Silver exert its lethal effects, even at low concentrations. Research suggests that most pathogenic organisms are killed in vitro at concentrations of 10 to 40 parts per million (ppm), with particularly sensitive organisms susceptible to 60 ppm.[71]

The development of nanochemistry has facilitated the production of microfine particles that increase silver's solubility and the release of silver ions in concentrations of 70 to 100 ppm.[72,73] Several sustained-silver dressings are available. Although these dressings differ in the technology used, as well as the characteristics of silver release, all are able to release more than the 10 to 40 ppm needed to achieve antisepsis.[72] Resistance to antiseptics is not a common problem. Data concerning the toxicity of silver ions are derived from what has been the experience with silver sulfadiazine. Silver absorption through intact skin is minimal; however, in full-thickness wounds, absorption of silver sulfadiazine may be as high as 10%.[72] Silver absorbed by epidermal cells induces the production of metallotheine, which, in turn, increases the uptake of zinc and copper and is postulated to increase RNA and DNA synthesis; this may promote cell proliferation and tissue repair.[71,74] Silver that is absorbed systemically may be found in the liver, brain, kidney, and bone marrow with apparently little toxic risk. Silver absorbed into the skin may cause argyria, which is a permanent dispigmentation of the skin; however, it is not life threatening.[72] There is some concern about the effect of silver on the proliferating cells in the bone marrow because there have been reports of neutropenia in children who were treated with silver sulfadiazine. White blood cell counts returned to normal when silver sulfadiazine was withheld; however, this is a sensitizing agent, and patients who developed leukopenia in the past should not be treated with silver again.[71] There has been a paucity of clinical trials evaluating the clinical efficacy of silver; thus, no strong conclusions may be drawn regarding this.

In summary, these dressings are useful tools in controlling the bacterial burden in wounds, but they may have cytotoxic effects and their judicious use is important.

MATRIX METALLOPROTEINASES AND THEIR INHIBITORS

Controlled degradation and formation of the ECM are an essential step in wound healing. This facilitates angiogenesis, migration of keratinocytes, reepithelialization, and remodeling of the provisional matrix. In addition, the ECM contains growth factors and cytokines that must be released to be activated. The turnover and remodeling of the ECM is tightly regulated.[1,75] The matrix metalloproteinases (MMPs) are a zinc-dependent group of enzymes that are capable of breaking down the major components of the ECM.[1,75] The production/activation of MMPs are regulated in three ways. First, it is regulated at the level of gene transcription, and this is induced by inflammatory cytokines and growth factors. Next, the enzymes are secreted as a zymogen and require activation by proteinases. Lastly, it is inhibited by another group of enzymes: the tissue inhibitors of metalloproteinases (TIMPs) and plasma α macroglobulin.[75] MMPs are mostly soluble proteins, except for the membrane-bound metalloproteinase. TIMPs are able to inhibit all unbound MMPs. TIMPs have cell growth–promoting, antiapoptotic, and antiangiogenic activity.[76] The generation of genetically engineered knock-out and transgenic mice provided vital information on the physiologic and pathologic functions of MMPs. Mice that lacked MMP-3 showed impaired dermal wound contraction, whereas mice lacking MMP-2 showed impaired angiogenesis. The most severe wound repair defect was seen in mice without MMP-7.[1] Conversely, the overexpression of MMP-1 by transgenic mice results in a hyperproliferative, hyperkeratotic epidermal phenotype and delayed wound closure.[77] MMPs seem to have overlapping substrate specificities and expression patterns. In healing wounds, MMPs follow a well-defined temporal and spatial profile. MMPs generally are not detected in normal intact skin; however, upon injury, MMP-1 is up-regulated, and its levels persist during healing and decrease with reepithelialization. MMP-1 is expressed in the advancing wound edge, whereas MMP-3 is found in the premigratory basal keratinocytes.[78,79] MMP-2 and -9 degrade the basement membrane and allow capillaries to form. In addition, MMPs are capable of cleaving and releasing inflammatory cytokines and interleukins and are responsible for releasing ECM-bound growth factors. MMPs are present in excessive amounts in chronic wounds, and their temporal pattern of expression is altered. Recent work by Nwomeh and colleagues[80] showed that chronic, nonhealing ulcers are characterized by significantly higher levels of MMP-1 and -8 and low levels of TIMP-1. Collagenases are in their inactive forms in normal healing wounds, whereas the activated enzyme is present at high concentrations in chronic ulcers. MMP-1, -2, -8, -9, and -14 were elevated in diabetic foot ulcers, whereas TIMP-2 was decreased.[81] MMP-9 was elevated in venous ulcers, and its levels correlated with poor healing. An elevated ratio of MMP-9/TIMP-1 also was related to nonhealing.[82] In summary, this altered expression of MMPs and TIMPs leads to persistent inflammation and excessive degradation of the ECM and growth factors.

What can we do to restore the balance of these enzymes in the chronic wound bed in the context of WBP? So far, attempts to target MMPs to produce healing in chronic wounds have not been successful. Because active MMPs are found in wound fluid, the therapeutic approach has been to develop dressings that could bind metalloproteinases and deactivate them. A collagen and oxidized regenerated cellulose dressing was formulated for this purpose. In vitro, Cullen and colleagues[83] showed that this dressing was able to decrease the in vitro activity of MMPs in wound fluid from nine patients. A randomized, double-blind clinical trial in diabetic ulcers showed no significant difference in the incidence of wound closure with this dressing and moistened gauze.[84] Targeting MMPs to improve wound healing is difficult because MMPs are essential to wound healing; however, they have to be present in the right amount and at the right time. Thus, nonspecific inhibition of MMPs is not a beneficial approach. Current areas of research are the development of selective MMP inhibitors; MMP modulation by using anti–tumor necrosis factor α medications;[85] and the use of activated protein C, which reduces inflammation and MMP production by inflammatory cells, but selectively stimulates MMP-2.[86] It is unlikely that medications that address the imbalance of MMPs in chronic wounds will solve the problem entirely; however, we will see more of these strategies in the future.

GROWTH FACTORS

Growth factors are polypeptides that act in concert in wound healing. Recent research using genetically engineered mice confirmed the expression of multiple growth factors and their receptors in different cell types of healing wounds. In addition, high levels and activation of growth factors during the healing process may facilitate wound closure. Growth factors have a characteristic spatial and temporal regulation; changes in this expression pattern bring about impaired healing.[2] The impaired function of one growth factor likely affects several growth factors and other cytokines. Also, there is a significant overlap in the functions of these growth factors.

The use of growth factors as therapeutic agents in chronic ulcers is the result of previous work that showed that the amount of these growth factors is decreased markedly in chronic wounds, secondary to the presence of high concentrations of proteases.[60,87,88] Conversely, several studies showed that growth factors are present in appropriate amounts, but are trapped within the fibrin cuffs in the surrounding capillaries or are bound to the ECM.[89–91] The result of suboptimal concentrations of growth factors is that cells in the wound bed become arrested in the cell cycle. Multiple in vitro and animal studies have shown the beneficial effect of growth factors, such as platelet-derived growth factors (PDGFs), fibroblast growth factors, and granulocyte-macrophage colony-stimulating factor, in healing.[92–95] PDGF is approved for use in diabetic foot ulcers, as supported by several clinical trials that showed statistically significant results. In a recent study, using a retrospective cohort study, Margolis and colleagues[96] showed that the effectiveness of PDGF in clinical trials also was present in clinical practice. The clinical data on the use of other growth factors have been mixed. Clinical trials of exogenous application of these growth factors failed to produce expected significant results. Currently, the focus of research on this treatment is to improve the delivery system to provide high concentrations to the wound bed or a more intimate relationship with the target cells. Gene therapy studies using adenoviral vectors are being conducted. In the future, the best results might be derived by using several growth factors that are specific for different stages of wound healing.

CELLULAR SENESCENCE OR NEAR SENESCENCE

The realization that the resident cells in chronic ulcers are phenotypically altered and exhibit senescence is a new concept. The efficacy of advanced treatments, such as growth factors and bioengineered skin, is dependent on the ability of these modalities to restore cellular competency in the wound bed.[97] The capacity of resident cells in the wound bed to replicate is critical to wound healing. Fibroblasts in chronic wounds display a senescent or a near-senescent phenotype. Senescent fibroblasts also exhibit a decreased mitogenic response to growth factors attributed to an abnormality in cell-signaling pathways. Chronic wound fibroblasts also produce elevated levels of proteolytic enzymes and decreased TIMPs. An important concept in cellular senescence is that cellular senescence is irreversible.[97] Thus, the continued exposure of cells in the wound bed to inflammatory cytokines, reactive oxygen species, and bacterial toxins results in an accumulation of senescent cells. It is postulated that when this population reaches a critical number, wounds are unlikely to heal, even with optimal care.[98]

Current treatment strategies to circumvent this problem are to remove senescent cells and repopulate the wound bed with viable nonsenescent fibroblasts by using tissue-engineered skin.[99,100] In vitro, it was shown that these products could counteract the inhibitory effects of wound exudate, possibly by delivery of growth factors in the correct temporal sequence and adequate concentration.[100] Other sources of nonsenescent fibroblasts are the wound margins and if quiescent fibroblasts could be induced to proliferate.[97] Because a substantial number of patients (up to 50%) are unresponsive to treatment, despite available advanced treatments, the search for new and effective strategies goes on.

The use of stem cells provides a promising rational therapeutic approach for chronic wounds. The ethical concerns regarding embryonic stem cell research have forced scientists to find more acceptable sources of these cells. Adult autologous bone marrow stem cells are a potential source of stem cells. These cells have unlimited replicative potential, differentiate into different tissues, and may provide needed cytokines and growth factors into the wound bed. Pilot studies have shown the great potential of this treatment; however, validation by randomized, clinical trials is needed.[101,102]

MONITORING PROGRESS IN WOUND HEALING

The ultimate goal of WBP is to achieve complete healing of the wound. One does not expect healing of chronic ulcers to occur overnight. Therefore, there needs to be a way to evaluate the progress of these wounds and to be assured that they are on their way to closure. A 15% decrease in wound area weekly has been suggested as the goal of treatment. Recently, a wound bed score that has a predictive value in wound closure was validated.[15] This wound bed score takes into account assessments of the wound bed as well as surrounding tissue that reflect the goals of adequate WBP (**Fig. 3**). Each

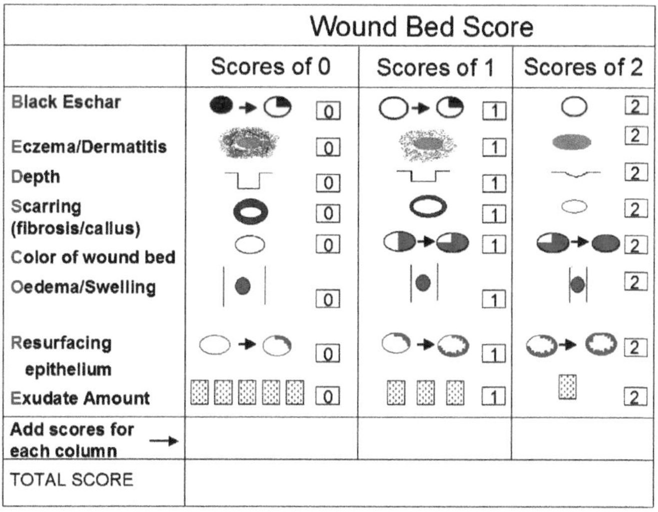

Fig. 3. Wound bed score and its individual features. The individual score for each characteristic is added to give a total wound bed score. The descriptors in parentheses below represent scores of 0, 1, and 2 points, respectively. Percentage of black eschar present (>25%, 1%–25%, 0%); severity of peri-ulcer eczema/dermatitis (severe, moderate, none or mild); depth of the wound (severely depressed or raised compared to peri-wound skin); severity of scarring (severe, moderate, none or minimal); percentage of pink-colored granulation tissue present (<50%, 50%–75%, >75%); severity of edema/swelling (severe, moderate, none/mild); percentage of regenerating epithelium (healing edges) (<25%, 25%–75%, >75%); severity of exudate/frequency of dressing changes (severe, moderate, none/mild). (*Courtesy of* V. Falanga, MD, Boston, MA. Copyright © 2007.)

parameter receives a score of 0 to 2, which is added to obtain the total score. The scores are divided into four quartiles: 4 to 9, 10 to 11, 12, and 13 to 16. With an increase in the wound bed score from one unit to the next (eg, from 10 to 13), there is a 22.8% increase in the odds of healing. This wound bed score will be useful in assessments as a predictor of initial healing and possibly for monitoring adequate response to treatment, with the expectation of achieving quartile increases in the wound bed time.

SUMMARY

The prerequisites for effective therapies are that the wound bed has little necrotic burden, a manageable bacterial load, minimal inflammation, and resident cells that can regenerate needed tissue. Thus, proper WBP is the first step toward achieving healing in the chronic wound. Advances in our understanding of the underlying problems of impaired healing will bring forth new and innovative therapies. The wound bed score having a predictive value for healing is useful for monitoring progress in treatment or the need to reevaluate current treatment strategies.

REFERENCES

1. Xue M, Le NT, Jackson CJ. Targeting matrix metalloproteases to improve cutaneous wound healing. Expert Opin Ther Targets 2006;10(1):143–55.

2. Werner S, Grose R. Regulation of wound healing by growth factors and cytokines. Physiol Rev 2003;83(3):835–70.

3. Cole J, Isik F. Human genomics and microarrays: implications for the plastic surgeon. Plast Reconstr Surg 2002;110(3):849–58.

4. Brown PO, Botstein D. Exploring the new world of the genome with DNA microarrays. Nat Genet 1999;21(1 Suppl):33–7.

5. Iyer VR, Eisen MB, Ross DT, et al. The transcriptional program in the response of human fibroblasts to serum. Science 1999;283(5398):83–7.

6. Copland JA, Davies PJ, Shipley GL, et al. The use of DNA microarrays to assess clinical samples: the transition from bedside to bench to bedside. Recent Prog Horm Res 2003;58:25–53.

7. Tomic-Canic M, Brem H. Gene array technology and pathogenesis of chronic wounds. Am J Surg 2004;188(1A Suppl):67–72.

8. Falanga V. Wound bed preparation and the role of enzymes: a case for multiple actions of therapeutic agents. Wounds 2002;14(2):47–74.

9. Falabella AF. Debridement and wound bed preparation. Dermatol Ther 2006; 19(6):317–25.

10. Steed DL, Donohoe D, Webster MW, et al. Effect of extensive debridement and treatment on the healing of diabetic foot ulcers. Diabetic Ulcer Study Group. J Am Coll Surg 1996;183(1):61–4.

11. Hellgren L, Vincent J. Debridement: an essential step in wound healing. In: Westerhof W, editor. Leg ulcers: diagnosis and treatment. Amsterdam: Elsevier Science Publishers; 1993. p. 305–12.

12. Miller JM. The interaction of papain, urea, and water-soluble chlorophyll in a proteolytic ointment for infected wounds. Surgery 1958;43(6):939–48.

13. Bonn D. Maggot therapy: an alternative for wound infection. Lancet 2000; 356(9236):1174.

14. Wollina U, Liebold K, Schmidt WD, et al. Biosurgery supports granulation and debridement in chronic wounds–clinical data and remittance spectroscopy measurement. Int J Dermatol 2002;41(10):635–9.

15. Falanga V, Saap LJ, Ozonoff A. Wound bed score and its correlation with healing of chronic wounds. Dermatol Ther 2006;19(6):383–90.

16. Bowler PG. The 10(5) bacterial growth guideline: reassessing its clinical relevance in wound healing. Ostomy Wound Manage 2003;49(1):44–53.

17. White RJ, Cutting K, Kingsley A. Topical antimicrobials in the control of wound bioburden. Ostomy Wound Manage 2006;52(8):26–58.

18. Gardner SE, Frantz RA, Doebbeling BN. The validity of the clinical signs and symptoms used to identify localized chronic wound infection. Wound Repair Regen 2001;9(3):178–86.

19. Dow G, Browne A, Sibbald RG. Infection in chronic wounds: controversies in diagnosis and treatment. Ostomy Wound Manage 1999;45(8):23–7, 29–40; quiz 41–22.

20. Cooper R. Understanding wound infection. In: Calnie S, editor. European Wound Management Association. Position document: identifying criteria for wound infection. London: Mep Ltd; 2005. p. 2–5.

21. Bowler PG, Duerden BI, Armstrong DG. Wound microbiology and associated approaches to wound management. Clin Microbiol Rev 2001;14(2): 244–69.

22. White RJ, Cutting KF. Critical colonization–the concept under scrutiny. Ostomy Wound Manage 2006;52(11):50–6.

23. Stephens P, Wall IB, Wilson MJ, et al. Anaerobic cocci populating the deep tissues of chronic wounds impair cellular wound healing responses in vitro. Br J Dermatol 2003;148(3):456–66.
24. Fuqua WC, Winans SC, Greenberg EP. Quorum sensing in bacteria: the LuxR-LuxI family of cell density-responsive transcriptional regulators. J Bacteriol 1994;176(2):269–75.
25. Ceri H, Olson ME, Stremick C, et al. The Calgary Biofilm Device: new technology for rapid determination of antibiotic susceptibilities of bacterial biofilms. J Clin Microbiol 1999;37(6):1771–6.
26. Mertz PM. Cutaneous biofilms: friend or foe? Wounds 2003;15:129–32.
27. Harrison-Balestra C, Cazzaniga AL, Davis SC, et al. A wound-isolated *Pseudomonas aeruginosa* grows a biofilm in vitro within 10 hours and is visualized by light microscopy. Dermatol Surg 2003;29(6):631–5.
28. Davies CE, Hill KE, Newcombe RG, et al. A prospective study of the microbiology of chronic venous leg ulcers to reevaluate the clinical predictive value of tissue biopsies and swabs. Wound Repair Regen 2007;15(1):17–22.
29. Levine NS, Lindberg RB, Mason AD Jr, et al. The quantitative swab culture and smear: a quick, simple method for determining the number of viable aerobic bacteria on open wounds. J Trauma 1976;16(2):89–94.
30. Armstrong DG, Liswood PJ, Todd WF. 1995 William J. Stickel Bronze Award. Prevalence of mixed infections in the diabetic pedal wound. A retrospective review of 112 infections. J Am Podiatr Med Assoc 1995;85(10):533–7.
31. Bornside GH, Bornside BB. Comparison between moist swab and tissue biopsy methods for quantitation of bacteria in experimental incisional wounds. J Trauma 1979;19(2):103–5.
32. Thomson PD, Smith DJ Jr. What is infection? Am J Surg 1994;167(1A):7S–10S [discussion: 10S–1S].
33. Lawrence JC. The bacteriology of burns. J Hosp Infect 1985;6(Suppl B):3–17.
34. Vindenes H, Bjerknes R. Microbial colonization of large wounds. Burns 1995; 21(8):575–9.
35. Bowler PG, Davies BJ. The microbiology of infected and noninfected leg ulcers. Int J Dermatol 1999;38(8):573–8.
36. Sapico FL, Witte JL, Canawati HN, et al. The infected foot of the diabetic patient: quantitative microbiology and analysis of clinical features. Rev Infect Dis 1984; 6(Suppl 1):S171–6.
37. Howell-Jones RS, Wilson MJ, Hill KE, et al. A review of the microbiology, antibiotic usage and resistance in chronic skin wounds. J Antimicrob Chemother 2005;55(2):143–9.
38. Bendy RH Jr, Nuccio PA, Wolfe E, et al. Relationship of quantitative wound bacterial counts to healing of decubiti: effect of topical gentamicin. Antimicrobial Agents Chemother (Bethesda) 1964;10:147–55.
39. Robson MC, Heggers JP. Bacterial quantification of open wounds. Mil Med 1969;134(1):19–24.
40. Robson MC, Heggers JP. Delayed wound closure based on bacterial counts. J Surg Oncol 1970;2(4):379–83.
41. Robson MC, Lea CE, Dalton JB, et al. Quantitative bacteriology and delayed wound closure. Surg Forum 1968;19:501–2.
42. Raahave D, Friis-Moller A, Bjerre-Jepsen K, et al. The infective dose of aerobic and anaerobic bacteria in postoperative wound sepsis. Arch Surg 1986;121(8): 924–9.

43. Majewski W, Cybulski Z, Napierala M, et al. The value of quantitative bacteriological investigations in the monitoring of treatment of ischaemic ulcerations of lower legs. Int Angiol 1995;14(4):381–4.
44. Trengove NJ, Stacey MC, McGechie DF, et al. Qualitative bacteriology and leg ulcer healing. J Wound Care 1996;5(6):277–80.
45. Kingston D, Seal DV. Current hypotheses on synergistic microbial gangrene. Br J Surg 1990;77(3):260–4.
46. Annoni F, Rosina M, Chiurazzi D, et al. The effects of a hydrocolloid dressing on bacterial growth and the healing process of leg ulcers. Int Angiol 1989;8(4):224–8.
47. Gilchrist B, Reed C. The bacteriology of chronic venous ulcers treated with occlusive hydrocolloid dressings. Br J Dermatol 1989;121(3):337–44.
48. Handfield-Jones SE, Grattan CE, Simpson RA, et al. Comparison of a hydrocolloid dressing and paraffin gauze in the treatment of venous ulcers. Br J Dermatol 1988;118(3):425–7.
49. Hansson C, Hoborn J, Moller A, et al. The microbial flora in venous leg ulcers without clinical signs of infection. Repeated culture using a validated standardised microbiological technique. Acta Derm Venereol 1995;75(1):24–30.
50. Sapico FL, Ginunas VJ, Thornhill-Joynes M, et al. Quantitative microbiology of pressure sores in different stages of healing. Diagn Microbiol Infect Dis 1986; 5(1):31–8.
51. Saap L, Fahim S, Arsenault E, et al. Contact sensitivity in patients with leg ulcerations: a North American study. Arch Dermatol 2004;140(10):1241–6.
52. Fraki JE, Peltonen L, Hopsu-Havu VK. Allergy to various components of topical preparations in stasis dermatitis and leg ulcer. Contact Dermatitis 1979;5(2): 97–100.
53. Eron LJ, Lipsky BA, Low DE, et al. Managing skin and soft tissue infections: expert panel recommendations on key decision points. J Antimicrob Chemother 2003;52(Suppl 1):i3–17.
54. Leaper DJ. Silver dressings: their role in wound management. Int Wound J 2006; 3(4):282–94.
55. Winter GD. Formation of the scab and the rate of epithelization of superficial wounds in the skin of the young domestic pig. Nature 1962;193:293–4.
56. Hinman CD, Maibach H. Effect of air exposure and occlusion on experimental human skin wounds. Nature 1963;200:377–8.
57. Drinkwater SL, Smith A, Sawyer BM, et al. Effect of venous ulcer exudates on angiogenesis in vitro. Br J Surg 2002;89(6):709–13.
58. Bucalo B, Eaglstein WH, Falanga V. Inhibition of cell proliferation by chronic wound fluid. Wound Repair Regen 1993;1(3):181–6.
59. Wysocki AB, Staiano-Coico L, Grinnell F. Wound fluid from chronic leg ulcers contains elevated levels of metalloproteinases MMP-2 and MMP-9. J Invest Dermatol 1993;101(1):64–8.
60. Trengove NJ, Stacey MC, MacAuley S, et al. Analysis of the acute and chronic wound environments: the role of proteases and their inhibitors. Wound Repair Regen 1999;7(6):442–52.
61. Grinnell F, Ho CH, Wysocki A. Degradation of fibronectin and vitronectin in chronic wound fluid: analysis by cell blotting, immunoblotting, and cell adhesion assays. J Invest Dermatol 1992;98(4):410–6.
62. Palfreyman SJ, Nelson EA, Lochiel R, et al. Dressings for healing venous leg ulcers. Cochrane Database Syst Rev 2006;3:CD001103.
63. Bolton LL, Monte K, Pirone LA. Moisture and healing: beyond the jargon. Ostomy Wound Manage 2000;46(1A Suppl):51S–62S, quiz 63S–4S.

64. Field FK, Kerstein MD. Overview of wound healing in a moist environment. Am J Surg 1994;167(1A):2S–6S.
65. Bolton LL, Johnson CL, Van Rijswijk L. Occlusive dressings: therapeutic agents and effects on drug delivery. Clin Dermatol 1991;9(4):573–83.
66. Akiyama H, Oono T, Saito M, et al. Assessment of cadexomer iodine against *Staphylococcus aureus* biofilm in vivo and in vitro using confocal laser scanning microscopy. J Dermatol 2004;31(7):529–34.
67. Chaw KC, Manimaran M, Tay FE. Role of silver ions in destabilization of intermo-lecular adhesion forces measured by atomic force microscopy in *Staphylococcus epidermidis* biofilms. Antimicrob Agents Chemother 2005;49(12):4853–9.
68. Lawrence JC. The use of iodine as an antiseptic agent. J Wound Care 1998;7(8):421–5.
69. Zhou LH, Nahm WK, Badiavas E, et al. Slow release iodine preparation and wound healing: in vitro effects consistent with lack of in vivo toxicity in human chronic wounds. Br J Dermatol 2002;146(3):365–74.
70. Lansdown AB. A review of the use of silver in wound care: facts and fallacies. Br J Nurs 2004;13(6 Suppl):S6–19.
71. Lansdown AB. Silver in health care: antimicrobial effects and safety in use. Curr Probl Dermatol 2006;33:17–34.
72. Lansdown AB, Williams A. How safe is silver in wound care? J Wound Care 2004;13(4):131–6.
73. Lansdown AB, Williams A, Chandler S, et al. Silver absorption and antibacterial efficacy of silver dressings. J Wound Care 2005;14(4):155–60.
74. Lansdown AB. Metallothioneins: potential therapeutic aids for wound healing in the skin. Wound Repair Regen 2002;10(3):130–2.
75. Ravanti L, Kahari VM. Matrix metalloproteinases in wound repair (review). Int J Mol Med 2000;6(4):391–407.
76. Will H, Atkinson SJ, Butler GS, et al. The soluble catalytic domain of membrane type 1 matrix metalloproteinase cleaves the propeptide of progelatinase A and initiates autoproteolytic activation. Regulation by TIMP-2 and TIMP-3. J Biol Chem 1996;271(29):17119–23.
77. Di Colandrea T, Wang L, Wille J, et al. Epidermal expression of collagenase delays wound-healing in transgenic mice. J Invest Dermatol 1998;111(6):1029–33.
78. Saarialho-Kere UK, Kovacs SO, Pentland AP, et al. Cell-matrix interactions modulate interstitial collagenase expression by human keratinocytes actively involved in wound healing. J Clin Invest 1993;92(6):2858–66.
79. Vaalamo M, Weckroth M, Puolakkainen P, et al. Patterns of matrix metalloprotei-nase and TIMP-1 expression in chronic and normally healing human cutaneous wounds. Br J Dermatol 1996;135(1):52–9.
80. Nwomeh BC, Liang HX, Diegelmann RF, et al. Dynamics of the matrix metallo-proteinases MMP-1 and MMP-8 in acute open human dermal wounds. Wound Repair Regen 1998;6(2):127–34.
81. Lobmann R, Ambrosch A, Schultz G, et al. Expression of matrix-metalloprotei-nases and their inhibitors in the wounds of diabetic and non-diabetic patients. Diabetologia 2002;45(7):1011–6.
82. Ladwig GP, Robson MC, Liu R, et al. Ratios of activated matrix metalloprotei-nase-9 to tissue inhibitor of matrix metalloproteinase-1 in wound fluids are inversely correlated with healing of pressure ulcers. Wound Repair Regen 2002;10(1):26–37.

83. Cullen B, Smith R, McCulloch E, et al. Mechanism of action of PROMOGRAN, a protease modulating matrix, for the treatment of diabetic foot ulcers. Wound Repair Regen 2002;10(1):16–25.

84. Veves A, Sheehan P, Pham HT. A randomized, controlled trial of Promogran (a collagen/oxidized regenerated cellulose dressing) vs standard treatment in the management of diabetic foot ulcers. Arch Surg 2002;137(7):822–7.

85. Taylor PC. Anti-TNFalpha therapy for rheumatoid arthritis: an update. Intern Med 2003;42(1):15–20.

86. Jackson CJ, Xue M, Thompson P, et al. Activated protein C prevents inflammation yet stimulates angiogenesis to promote cutaneous wound healing. Wound Repair Regen 2005;13(3):284–94.

87. Trengove NJ, Bielefeldt-Ohmann H, Stacey MC. Mitogenic activity and cytokine levels in non-healing and healing chronic leg ulcers. Wound Repair Regen 2000; 8(1):13–25.

88. Tarnuzzer RW, Schultz GS. Biochemical analysis of acute and chronic wound environments. Wound Repair Regen 1996;4(3):321–5.

89. Falanga V, Eaglstein WH. The "trap" hypothesis of venous ulceration. Lancet 1993;341(8851):1006–8.

90. Falanga V. Chronic wounds: pathophysiologic and experimental considerations. J Invest Dermatol 1993;100(5):721–5.

91. Higley HR, Ksander GA, Gerhardt CO, et al. Extravasation of macromolecules and possible trapping of transforming growth factor-beta in venous ulceration. Br J Dermatol 1995;132(1):79–85.

92. Edmonds M, Bates M, Doxford M, et al. New treatments in ulcer healing and wound infection. Diabetes Metab Res Rev 2000;16(Suppl 1):S51–4.

93. Greenhalgh DG. The role of growth factors in wound healing. J Trauma 1996; 41(1):159–67.

94. Harding KG, Morris HL, Patel GK. Science, medicine and the future: healing chronic wounds. BMJ 2002;324(7330):160–3.

95. Nath C, Gulati SC. Role of cytokines in healing chronic skin wounds. Acta Haematol 1998;99(3):175–9.

96. Margolis DJ, Bartus C, Hoffstad O, et al. Effectiveness of recombinant human platelet-derived growth factor for the treatment of diabetic neuropathic foot ulcers. Wound Repair Regen 2005;13(6):531–6.

97. Vande Berg JS, Robson MC. Arresting cell cycles and the effect on wound healing. Surg Clin North Am 2003;83(3):509–20.

98. Harding KG, Moore K, Phillips TJ. Wound chronicity and fibroblast senescence–implications for treatment. Int Wound J 2005;2(4):364–8.

99. Falanga V, Margolis D, Alvarez O, et al. Rapid healing of venous ulcers and lack of clinical rejection with an allogeneic cultured human skin equivalent. Human Skin Equivalent Investigators Group. Arch Dermatol 1998;134(3):293–300.

100. Veves A, Falanga V, Armstrong DG, et al. Graftskin, a human skin equivalent, is effective in the management of noninfected neuropathic diabetic foot ulcers: a prospective randomized multicenter clinical trial. Diabetes Care 2001;24(2): 290–5.

101. Cha J, Falanga V. Stem cells in cutaneous wound healing. Clin Dermatol 2007; 25(1):73–8.

102. Falanga V, Iwamoto S, Chartier M, et al. Autologous bone marrow-derived cultured mesenchymal stem cells delivered in a fibrin spray accelerate healing in murine and human cutaneous wounds. Tissue engineering 2007;13: 1299–312.

Suture Choice and Other Methods of Skin Closure

Julio Hochberg, MD*, Kathleen M. Meyer, MD, Michael D. Marion, MD

KEYWORDS

- Skin closure • Sutures • Surgical needles • Staples
- Topical adhesives • Tapes

Historically, there were few surgical options for wound closure. From catgut, silk, and cotton, there is now an ever-increasing array of sutures, approximately 5,269 different types, including antibiotic-coated and knotless sutures. In addition to the continual advancement in suture material, the variety and refinement of surgical needles and packaging has also increased. New closure methods have recently been developed, such as topical adhesives and absorbable staples, which can either be used alone or in combination with traditional suture repair.

The surgeon evaluating a skin laceration has to choose the best closure method for that particular patient and wound from a multitude of possibilities. Closing a wound in an infant differs greatly from closing a wound in an elderly patient with multiple comorbidities, such as diabetes, heart disease, steroids use, and thin skin. Skin itself varies throughout the body in terms of its thickness, elasticity, speed of healing, and tendency to scar. Suture techniques that avoid suture marks such as "railroad tracks," especially in skin exposed in normal clothing, are generally more aesthetically pleasing to the patient. In the selection of a suture, a patient's health status, age, weight and comfort, and the presence or absence of infection are as important as the biomechanical properties of the suture, individual wound characteristics,[1] anatomic location, and a surgeon's personal preference and experience in handling a suture material. There is often more than one appropriate method of closure. Although suture materials from different companies have similar chemical components, the performance and quality of these products are not always equivalent.

The ultimate responsibility for the choice of the best material lies with the surgeon. The cost of a complication, such as wound dehiscence, a fistula, reoperations, pain, and even death, will never justify the use of a less expensive, lower quality suture.

Choosing a method of closure that affords a technically easy and efficient procedure, with a secure closure and minimal pain and scaring, is paramount to any

Department of Surgery, Marshfield Clinic, 1000 North Oak Avenue, Marshfield, WI 54449, USA
* Corresponding author.
E-mail address: drhamburger@gmail.com (J. Hochberg).

Surg Clin N Am 89 (2009) 627–641
doi:10.1016/j.suc.2009.03.001
0039-6109/09/$ – see front matter © 2009 Elsevier Inc. All rights reserved.

surgeon. This article addresses the current state of affairs of sutures and methods of wound closure. The nuances, advantages and disadvantages, and strengths and weaknesses of various suture choices in different circumstances are reviewed. Much of this reflection is based on the collective experience of the authors, each of whom has trained at a different institution and brings a unique set of experiences to the discussion.

PROPERTIES OF SUTURE MATERIALS
Tensile Strength

Tensile strength is the measured force, in pounds, that the suture will withstand before it breaks.[2,3] Suture material should have, and maintain, adequate tensile strength for its specified purpose.[2]

Tissue Absorption

Tissue absorption is a suture characteristic distinct from the rate of tensile strength loss. A suture may display rapid loss of tensile strength yet be absorbed slowly.[4] An absorbable suture is defined as a suture that undergoes degradation and absorption in tissues. A nonabsorbable suture maintains its tensile strength and is resistant to absorption. However, most foreign materials will eventually undergo some degree of degradation over time. The rate of absorption is especially pertinent to late suture complications, such as the development of sinus tracts and granulomas.[5] Absorbable sutures are generally used for buried sutures that approximate deep tissues.[6] Nonabsorbable sutures are most commonly used externally in the skin and will eventually be removed, or for wounds in deeper structures that require prolonged support.[6] Factors that delay wound healing are many and include, but are not limited to, diabetes, corticosteroid therapy, malnutrition, stress, and systemic disease. Such factors significantly influence suture choice, and with an increased risk of delayed healing, a nonabsorbable external closure would likely be chosen over an absorbable suture.

Cross-Sectional Diameter

Suture diameter designations are specified in descending sequence (ie, 1-0 is larger than 11-0). When selecting suture size, the finest gauge commensurate with the natural strength of the tissue is recommended.[3] The number and diameter of sutures used to close a wound should be the minimum necessary for coaptation of the edges.

Coefficient of Friction

The coefficient of friction pertains to how easily a suture passes through tissue.[4]

Knot Security

Knot strength is calculated by determining the force necessary to cause a knot to slip.[4,7] The least reliable part of any suture is the knot.[3] Knot security is the quality of a suture that allows it to be tied securely with a minimum number of throws per knot.[2] Greater knot strength minimizes the risk of wound dehiscence. A knot stays tied because of the friction produced by one part of the knot acting on another, which relates to the coefficient of friction of the suture material. A suture with a high coefficient of friction has good knot security but tends to abrade and drag through tissue.[8] A knot should hold securely without fraying or cutting. For safety, a knot should have at least 3 throws with 3-mm long ends. Smooth surfaces decrease knot security and must be compensated for with extra throws.

Elasticity

Elasticity is the ability of a material to return to its original length after stretching.[4] High elasticity will allow the suture to stretch with wound edema but return to its original length and form once swelling has subsided. A high degree of elasticity provides obvious clinical advantages, because highly elastic suture material is less likely to cut through the skin with swelling and effectively approximates wound edges throughout the healing process.

Plasticity

Plasticity is defined as the capacity of a suture to be permanently molded or altered.[4] Plasticity refers to the ability of a suture to stretch with wound edema without return to its original form once swelling subsides. Thus, sutures that are highly plastic may become too loose when swelling decreases and fail to correctly appose wound edges.

Memory

Memory is the capacity of a suture to assume a stable linear configuration after removal from packaging and after stretching. Memory is the capacity of a suture to remain free of curling and other contortions that may interfere with surgical handling and use. Sutures with significant memory are not pliable, which makes them difficult to work with, and significant memory necessitates additional knots.[9] (Nylon has significant memory, whereas Gore-Tex suture has no memory).

Handling

Several factors impact on how a suture handles including elasticity, plasticity, and memory.[3] The material should handle comfortably and naturally. The hallmark of silk is its exceptional handling characteristics (workability) and ease of knot tying, setting the standard with which all other material is compared.[3,6]

Tissue Reactivity

All suture materials are foreign to human tissue and may elicit a tissue reaction,[3] such as an inflammatory response, that interferes with wound healing and increases the risk of infection. The duration and severity of the tissue response depends on the type and quantity of suture material used along with its configuration.[9,10] An ideal suture stimulates minimal tissue reaction and does not create a situation favorable to bacterial growth. Suture material should be nonelectrolytic, noncapillary, nonallergenic, and noncarcinogenic.

Origin

Suture material may be either natural or synthetic; natural fibers (eg, surgical gut and silk) cause a more intense inflammatory reaction than synthetic material (eg, polypropylene).

Physical Configuration

Suture material may be composed either of a single filament or multiple filaments.

- *Monofilament.* Monofilament sutures have several desirable qualities, including strength, low tissue drag, and low propensity to harbor infection. The incidence of wound infection is significantly lower with monofilament compared with braided sutures.[4,11] However, monofilament sutures do not handle as easily as braided sutures.

- *Multifilament (braided or twisted).* A multifilament configuration handles easily but has been shown to promote tissue infection and reactivity.[2] The increase in tissue infection is a result of capillary penetration by bacteria and other foreign materials. A braided suture may harbor bacteria within its crevices and bacteria may escape phagocytosis.[4,12]

Capillarity

Capillarity of a suture describes the ease of transporting liquids along the suture strand and is an inherent physical property of multifilament sutures due to the available interstitial space. Capillarity is related to the ability of a suture to transport and spread microorganisms and is an important property in terms of wound infection. A braided nylon could take up to three times as many microorganisms as monofilament nylon. Monofilament sutures do not exhibit capillarity. Braided polyester (Mersilene) shows capillarity, whereas braided silk with wax and plain and chromic gut do not have capillarity.[13]

Fluid Absorption

Fluid absorption and capillarity properties are presumed to be of significance due to the impact of contaminating bacteria on tissues. The chemical nature and physical structure of sutures determine the level of fluid absorption. However, the chemical nature seems to be more important than the physical structure. Synthetic sutures have much lower fluid absorption capability than natural sutures, because synthetic sutures are more hydrophobic. Multifilament sutures have a higher fluid absorption than monofilament sutures. Plain and chromic gut sutures demonstrate the highest fluid absorption.[13]

Ease of Removal

For wounds from which suture removal may be painful or difficult and support is only needed for a short time period, rapidly absorbable sutures are indicated.

Color

Sutures are available in dyed and undyed material. A dyed material provides easy visualization when the sutures are removed. If suture removal is not planned, undyed material can be used to avoid unsightly show through the skin.

SUTURES
Absorbable

- *Polyglactic 910 (Vicryl)* is a synthetic, absorbable, braided suture made of polyglactin 910 coated with a copolymer of L-lactide and glycolide (Polyglactin 370) and calcium stearate. Polyglactic 910 thus retains 65% of its tensile strength at 2 weeks and 40% at 3 weeks. It is extremely useful as a completely buried suture to approximate wound edges until the wound has gained enough strength to keep the edges from separating.[6] Complete absorption of Vicryl occurs between 60 and 90 days by hydrolysis. There is less of an inflammatory response due to the absorption of polyglactic acid by hydrolysis if compared with the proteolytic absorption of surgical gut.[2] Vicryl is available in a clear undyed or violet-dyed form. In cutaneous closures, the dyed form is often visible beneath the skin surface. Vicryl can be extruded if used in the subcuticular layer.
- *Polyglactic 910 (Vicryl Rapide)* is a synthetic, absorbable, multifilament suture. It is derived from polyglactin 910 that is partially hydrolyzed in a buffer solution and sterilized with gamma irradiation. This processing speeds absorption, leaving the

mechanical properties of the suture intact.[14] Fifty percent of tensile strength is retained at 5 days. At 2 weeks, the tensile strength is 0%. *Vicryl Rapide* sutures fall off in 10 to 14 days and absorption occurs by hydrolysis in 7 to 14 days.

- *Antibacterial suture (coated Vicryl Plus)* is an absorbable suture with an antimicrobial coating that was first developed using triclosan, a well-known antimicrobial material with a long history of safe use as the active agent in consumer health care products.[4] Pediatric surgeons noted less postoperative pain in patients treated with coated Vicryl Plus. The reduction in postoperative pain was attributed to inhibition of bacterial colonization and, likely, the avoidance of subclinical infection.[15] Long-term studies are not yet available.

- *Polyglycolic suture (Dexon II)* is a synthetic, coated, braided, absorbable suture made of polyglycolic acid polycaprolate. The lubricant coating decreases the coefficient of friction. Polyglycolic acid retains 89% of its tensile strength at 7 days, 63% at 14 days, and 17% at 21 days.[16] Compared with Dexon, Vicryl showed the slowest loss of function and the highest knot-breaking strength. In the same study, Dexon II showed the greatest irreversible elongation.[17]

- *Poliglecaprone (Monocryl)* is a synthetic, absorbable, monofilament suture made of a copolymer of glycolide and e-capralactone. In a side-by-side comparison with Vicryl Rapide, poliglecarpone subcuticular closure resulted in significantly smaller, less reactive scars and a lower tendency to hypertrophic scar formation.[18] This suture has significant initial tensile strength, which allows for the selection of a suture that is 1 to 2 sizes smaller than would customarily be chosen.[4] Dyed Monocryl retains 30 to 40% of its tensile strength at 2 weeks, whereas undyed Monocryl retains 25% at 2 weeks and 0% at 21 days. Absorption of the sutures occurs by hydrolysis in approximately 90 to 120 days.

- *Polydioxanone (PDS)* is a synthetic, absorbable, monofilament suture made from polyester, poly(*p*-dioxanone). This suture retains 74% of its tensile strength after 2 weeks, 50% after 4 weeks and 25% after 6 weeks. Polydioxanone is somewhat stiff and difficult to handle. It is a low reactivity suture that maintains its integrity in the presence of bacterial infection.[6] The absorption rate of this material is minimal until 90 days and it is absorbed slowly by hydrolysis in 180 to 210 days.

- *Polyglycolide-trimethylene carbonate (Maxon)* is a synthetic, absorbable, monofilament suture. It is a copolymer of glycolide and trimethylene carbonate. Compared with PDS, Maxon was somewhat unwieldy.[19] Maxon can be used for the deep and superficial portions of a closure. Tensile strength was measurable for 42 to 92 days for Maxon, and 64 to 80 days for PDS. Absorption of Maxon is complete in 6 to 7 months.[4]

- *Barbed suture (Quill SRS)* is a knotless, synthetic suture made of dyed polydioxanone and is now available as undyed polyglecaprone (Monoderm). Barbed suture is effective due to bidirectional fixation within the wound. Closure with barbed sutures begins at the midpoint of the wound with suturing that extends in two directions from the midpoint. Barbs within the suture distribute tension across the wound and eliminate the need for knots.[20] This material facilitates the use of a continuous suturing technique in place of interrupted sutures in a deep, layered closure. Because the Quill suture cannot slip backward, it does not gap in areas of tension, allowing an esthetic subcuticular closure with fewer preliminary buried sutures, which affords significant time savings (as much as one half to two thirds). Thus, the greatest benefit of using

Quill suture is its speed in closing deep layers. However, a disadvantage is that this suture has significant memory, and the needle size is not always appropriate for certain procedures. The product is in its infancy and will surely be refined.

- *Plain, chromic and fast-absorbing plain gut* are biologic, absorbable, monofilament sutures. These materials are made by twisting together strands of mostly purified collagen prepared from the submucosal layers of the small intestine of sheep or the serosal layer of the small intestine of cattle. The plain gut is untreated, the strength retention is 7 days, and absorption occurs in 10 to 14 days. The chromic gut is tanned with chromic salts to increase the holding time to approximately 14 days with absorption in 21 days. Fast-absorbing plain gut is heat-treated to create more rapid absorption. These sutures have less tensile strength than plain gut of comparable size. Fast-absorbing plain gut is used primarily for epidermal suturing where sutures are required for only 5 to 7 days. Fast-absorbing plain gut is helpful for suturing wounds in children or wounds in locations from which it is difficult to remove sutures.[2] Chromic gut is absorbed by proteolysis and macrophages, and plain gut attracts small lymphocytes that facilitate absorption.[21,22]

Nonabsorbable

- *Nylon (Ethilon)*, a synthetic, nonabsorbable, monofilament suture made of a chemically inert polyamide polymer fiber, has low tissue reactivity. Nylon sutures are the most commonly used sutures in cutaneous operations.[6] The tensile strength of this material at 2 weeks is high, with a potential loss of 50% by 1 to 2 years due to progressive hydrolysis over time.
- *Polypropylene (Prolene)*, a synthetic, nonabsorbable, monofilament suture made by catalytic polymerization of propylene, has low tissue reactivity and high tensile strength, similar to nylon. Polypropylene has as an extremely smooth surface, which decreases knot security and must be compensated for with extra throws. A significant advantage of Prolene is its high plasticity, and ability to accommodate wound edema. Polypropylene is easy to remove and is therefore an ideal suture for a running, subcuticular stitch.[6] This suture is also not subject to degradation.
- *Silk* is a natural, nonabsorbable, braided suture that is white, extruded by silk worm larvae, and made of protein filaments. Surgical silk is braided for easy handling and dyed for greater visibility. Silk has good knot security but evokes a significant inflammatory response. Owing to its braided configuration, silk is also prone to infection and can be infiltrated by tissue ingrowth. Silk suffers progressive degradation that may result in gradual loss of tensile strength.
- *Braided polyester (Mersilene)* is a synthetic, nonabsorbable, uncoated, braided or monofilament suture material. The tensile strength at 2 weeks is high, and the material has a high coefficient of friction. The monofilament form has poor knot security, whereas the braided form gives a more secure knot. The braided form cannot be used in the presence of infection or contamination.[6] This suture has low tissue reactivity and undergoes no significant changes in vivo.
- *ePTFE (Gore-Tex CV4)* is a synthetic, nonabsorbable, monofilament suture made of polytetrafluoroethylene that has been expanded to produce a porous microstructure that is 50% air by volume. This suture is white in color and provokes minimal tissue response with cellular ingrowth. The tensile strength does not change in vivo. Gore-Tex is soft and supple, affording excellent handling.

Gore-Tex does not degrade in the presence of infection and is not subject to the action of tissue enzymes.

SURGICAL NEEDLES

Needles are manufactured from stainless steel wire, which has excellent resistance to corrosion. Needles are chosen based on strength, temper, rigidity, malleability, ductility, and surface finish. Needles must be matched to the patient and surgery. The factors to be considered include the thickness and accessibility of the tissue to be sutured, the importance of attaining a good cosmetic result, and the size of the suture material.[2] Surgical needle performance is determined by the following parameters: sharpness, resistance to bending, resistance to breaking (ductility), and by the force that must be exerted to grasp a curved needle with the jaws of the needle holder.[5] Surgical needles have distinctive anatomy and characteristics, such as shape, size, point, and method of suture attachment.

Needle Anatomy

- *Eye*: the eye is the site of attachment of the needle to the suture. The close eye is similar to a household sewing needle. The French eye has a slit from inside the eye to the end of the needle that holds the suture. The swaged needle is configured so that the suture and the needle form a continuous unit.
- *Body*: the body of the needle is the portion grasped by the needle holder.
- *Point*: the point of the needle extends from the tip to the maximum cross-sectional area of the body.

Needle Shape

- *1/4 circle*: used in microsurgery.
- *3/8 circle*: used to approximate the divided edges of thin planar structures that are readily accessible (ie, skin).
- *1/2 circle*: used in deep body cavities and other confined locations.
- *5/8 circle*: used in the nasal cavity.
- *1/2 curved or ski*: used in endoscopic procedures.
- *Straight*: used when suturing easily accessible tissue, where direct finger-held manipulation can be easily performed.

Needle Size

The choice of the length and curvature of a needle is determined by the size and depth of the wound. The diameter of the needle should match the suture size to minimize damage as the needle passes through tissue.

Needle Points

Each type of needle point is designed to penetrate a specific type of tissue. Needle points are either cut, tapered, or a combination of both.[3]

- *Conventional cutting*. The needle body is triangular and has two opposing cutting edges and a third edge on the inside of the curve. This configuration creates a track that faces the wound edge, producing the potential to accidentally cut tissue.[3] (This point is used in tough tissues like skin and mucosa.)
- *Reverse cutting*. This needle point has the third cutting edge on the outside of the curve to avoid the possibility of accidentally cutting tissue. (This point is used in tough tissues like skin, mucosa, and in the nasal cavity.)

- *Precision cosmetic.* This form offers the most honed point for maintaining sharpness. (This is used in delicate plastic or cosmetic surgery and on the skin.)
- *Trocar point or tapercut.* The needle body is round, tapered and ends in a small triangular cutting point. The cutting edges of the trocar point needle extend only a short distance from the needle tip and blend into a round, tapered body.[5] (This point is used for closures in the oral mucosa and nasal cavity.)
- *Spatula point.* This point is flat on the top and bottom with a cutting edge along the front to one side. (This point is used with corneal or scleral tissue.)
- *Blunt point.* This is simply a blunted, dull point. (This point is used for friable tissues such as fascia.)
- *Taper.* The needle body is round and tapers smoothly to a point that spreads the tissue without cutting it. (This point is used in soft tissue that does not resist needle penetration, such as fascia, subcutaneous fat, and muscle.)
- *Keith needle.* This is a straight, cutting needle. (This point is used primarily for skin closure of abdominal wounds.)
- *Specialty needles.* There are needle points especially designed for cleft palate and microsurgery.

SUTURE ATTACHMENT

- *Swaged needle* (atraumatic needle) provides a less traumatic, smaller diameter needle[3] that does not require preparation or handling. The needle may be permanently swaged to the suture or may be designed to come off with a sharp, straight tug. These "pop-offs" are commonly used for interrupted sutures, whereby each suture is only passed once and then tied.[5] Nearly all modern sutures feature the swaged, atraumatic needle.
- *Threaded needle* (traumatic needle) is a needle whereby the suture is threaded through the eye of the needle. Threaded needles are more difficult to handle and cause more tissue trauma than swaged needles. Threaded needles are rarely used today. However, a threaded needle may salvage a suture line if a continuous suture has broken.

SUTURING TECHNIQUES

- *Simple interrupted sutures.* These are the most commonly used sutures and are useful in linear or irregular wounds. The needle is introduced at a 90° angle into the skin to include a larger portion of the deeper dermis.[21] This method allows the width of the suture at its base in the dermis to be wider than the epidermal entrance and exit points.[6] An advantage of interrupted sutures is that more selective adjustments of wound edges can be made.[2]
- *Vertical mattress sutures.* These sutures are appropriate for either thick or thin skin. Vertical mattress sutures are used if eversion is not achieved with simple interrupted sutures. This suture provides a secure grasp of tissue and a good approximation of the skin margins. Vertical mattress sutures need to be soft and pliable but should not stretch tissue. These sutures help distribute tension. Unfortunately, permanent hatch mark scars result if the sutures are left in place for more than 5 to 7 days.[6,23]
- *Half buried horizontal mattress or 3-corner sutures.* This type of suture is used for flap edges, because the suture minimizes tissue ischemia. The 3-corner suture is especially useful for closing a V-shaped wound or for approximating skin edges that differ in texture or thickness.

- *Horizontal mattress*. This suture is useful in situations where compression of wound edges is necessary for hemostasis. The horizontal mattress suture may also be used to close wounds under moderate tension and to increase wound tensile strength during the period of wound healing. In addition, the horizontal mattress suture can be used to evert wound edges. However, this suture can lead to tissue ischemia and therefore must be applied loosely, which may make the wound appear untidy after the repair.
- *Horizontal continuous mattress.* These sutures are useful in everting wound edges in areas prone to inversion, such as the retroauricular skin.
- *Subcuticular continuous suture*. This suture provides an excellent way to achieve accurate skin edge apposition without external sutures or cross-hatching. The suture can be an absorbable suture, such as polyglactic 910 (Vicryl) or poligle-caprone (Monocryl), or a nonabsorbable suture, such as polypropylene (Prolene), with external knots that are easy to remove.[6]
- *Running continuous sutures*. The running continuous suture provides a rapid, secure closure with an even distribution of tension along the length of the wound preventing tightness in any one area. It is used for linear wounds. This technique also provides additional wound eversion. The only real disadvantage of the running continuous suture is demonstrated if the suture breaks or the surgeon wants to remove only a few sutures at a time.[2] Gaps can occur in any continuous suture method if the tension is not controlled with a deep closure.
- *Continuous locking suture*. These sutures are useful for suturing dermal matrix (*Alloderm*). However, the continuous locking suture leaves permanent hatch marks in the skin.
- *Purse-string sutures*. This is a continuous suture placed around a circle, such as the areola. This suture has the disadvantage of inverting tissues.
- *Buried sutures*. These sutures are placed so that the knot protrudes to the inside, under the layer to be closed.
- *Quilting sutures*. This suture refers to the attachment of a skin flap to the underlying aponeurosis with multiple sutures and is an efficient technique for prevention of seroma formation.[24]
- *Frost sutures*. These are suspension sutures used in eyelid surgery to prevent ectropium.
- *Figure-of-eight or far-near-far pulley suture*. These suture are a modification of the vertical mattress suture. The suture provides a pulley effect that allows wound closure under tension, such as the closure of the latissimus dorsi myocutaneous flap donor site. Figure-of-eight sutures have to be removed early to avoid cross-hatching.
- *Ligatures*. This is a suture tied around a vessel for hemostatic purposes.
- *Retention sutures*. Retention sutures have been used in an attempt to reduce the risk of acute fascial dehiscence and to repair postoperative fascial dehiscence. However, these sutures do not seem to reduce the risk of wound complications. In addition, in one study, 50% of patients with retention sutures had them removed prematurely due to pain.[12,25]

SUTURE KNOTS

Knots must be tight enough to coapt the wound edges and should be no tighter. Regarding knot strength, sliding knots with extra throws are as secure as square knots, and surgeon's knots are no more secure than square knots for smaller diameter sutures.[26] For safety, a knot should have at least three throws with 3-mm long ends. Smooth surfaces, as seen with monofilament sutures, decrease knot security and must be compensated for with extra throws.

PRINCIPLES OF SUTURING SKIN WOUNDS

1. The primary function of the suture is to maintain tissue approximation during healing.
2. Sutures placed in the dermal layer provide tensile strength, and control tension for the outer layer.
3. Sutures placed in the epidermis should coapt the edges and correct any intervening gaps in the suture line or discrepancies in height between the two sides.
4. Debridment of the skin edges should be done if necessary.
5. Avoidance of direct tissue trauma helps ensure optimal outcomes.[21]
6. Clean passage of the needle, following the arc, is imperative, as is avoidance of multiple punctures.[21]
7. Skin sutures that blanch the underlying skin are too tight.[21]
8. Skin edges are always kept everted and without tension. The everted skin edges will gradually flatten.
9. Skin edges must just touch each other.

SUTURES ACCORDING TO ANATOMIC LOCATION

The final decision concerning the method and material used in closure is highly dependent on the length and anatomic location of the wound (**Table 1**).[7,27,28]

STAPLES

- *Nonabsorbable (Proximate).* These staples are made of stainless steel and combine the highest tensile strength of any suture material in use today with a low tissue reactivity.[2] Metal staples come in two sizes, regular and wide, and are dispensed from lightweight easy to grip cartridges. Metal staples provide a faster closure than sutures.[2,29] Metal staples also provide excellent wound edge eversion without strangulation of tissue and result in minimal cross-hatch scarring.[23] Staples yield a satisfactory result for cutaneous wound closure in a wide variety of circumstances and are extremely useful in fixation of skin grafts. Metal staples may offer a slightly superior cosmetic outcome when used to close scalp wounds. It is common to use staples to close scalp wounds that are under a great deal of tension. Contaminated wounds closed with staples have a lower incidence of infection than those closed with sutures. Staple closure also eliminates the risk that a health care provider will experience a needle stick, which is a particularly important consideration in caring for trauma patients with unknown medical histories. There are specially designed extractors for staple removal, although removal can also be accomplished with a hemostat.
- *Absorbable (Insorb).* A novel form of skin closure that uses absorbable subcuticular staples is now available. The staple is composed of an absorbable copolymer of predominantly polylactide and a lesser component of polyglycolide.[30] The closure of contaminated wounds with Insorb staples was found to be superior to closure with Vicryl sutures, because the Insorb staples had a significantly lower incidence of infection.[4] Insorb staples will not interfere with MRI examinations. In some studies, the performance of Insorb staples was similar to that of percutaneous metal staples with respect to the development of wound infection.

Table 1
Suture choice according to anatomic location of wound

Anatomic Location	Tissue Layer	Options
Scalp	Dermal	4-0 Vicryl simple interrupted sutures
	Epidermal	5-0 Vicryl Rapide continuous running suture
		Metal staples or 4-0 Prolene simple interrupted sutures (1-layer closure)
Face	Dermal	5-0 Vicryl simple interrupted sutures
		5-0 Vicryl, 5-0 Monocryl or 5-0 Prolene continuous subcuticular suture
	Epidermal	6-0 Monocryl simple interrupted sutures
		6-0 Nylon or 6-0 fast-absorbing plain gut simple interrupted sutures or 6-0 Monocryl continuous running suture or Dermabond (1-layer closure)
Ears		
Anterior	Epidermal	6-0 Monocryl simple interrupted sutures
		6-0 Nylon simple interrupted sutures
Lobe	Dermal	5-0 Vicryl simple interrupted sutures
	Epidermal	6-0 Monocryl simple interrupted sutures
		6-0 Nylon simple interrupted sutures
Posterior	Epidermal	5-0 Monocryl continuous horizontal mattress suture
		5-0 Nylon continuous horizontal mattress suture
Lips	Muscle	5-0 Vicryl simple interrupted sutures
	Mucosa	5-0 Vicryl simple interrupted sutures
	Vermilion	6-0 Silk simple interrupted sutures
		6-0 Nylon or 6-0 Vicryl simple interrupted sutures
	Epidermal	6-0 Vicryl Rapide simple interrupted sutures
		6-0 Monocryl or 6-0 Nylon simple interrupted sutures
Eyelids	Epidermal	6-0 Monocryl continuous running suture
		6-0 Prolene continuous running suture or 6-0 Nylon simple interrupted sutures
Neck	Dermal	5-0 Vicryl simple interrupted sutures
		6-0 Vicryl, 6-0 Monocryl or 6-0 Prolene continuous subcuticular suture
	Epidermal	6-0 Monocryl continuous running suture

(continued on next page)

Table 1
(continued)

Anatomic Location	Tissue Layer	Options	
Breasts	Dermal	3-0 Vicryl simple interrupted sutures	4-0 Quill, 5-0 Vicryl, or 5-0 Prolene continuous subcuticular suture
	Epidermal	5-0 Monocryl continuous running suture	5-0 Nylon simple interrupted sutures
Areola	Dermal	4-0 Vicryl simple interrupted sutures	3-0 Gore-Tex CV4 pull-string sutures or 5-0 Vicryl simple interrupted sutures
	Epidermal	6-0 Monocryl continuous running suture	—
Presternal	Dermal	3-0 Vicryl simple interrupted sutures	—
	Epidermal	5-0 Monocryl continuous running suture	Metal staples
Abdomen	Dermal	3-0 Vicryl simple interrupted sutures	5-0 Monocryl or 5-0 Prolene continuous subcuticular suture
	Epidermal	4-0 Monocryl continuous running suture	Metal staples
Back	Dermal	3-0 Vicryl simple interrupted sutures	—
	Epidermal	4-0 Monocryl continuous running suture	5-0 Nylon simple interrupted sutures
Arm and forearm	Dermal	4-0 Vicryl simple interrupted sutures	—
	Epidermal	5-0 Monocryl continuous running suture	5-0 Nylon simple interrupted sutures
Hand	Epidermal	5-0 Nylon simple interrupted sutures	—
Palm	Epidermal	5-0 Nylon simple interrupted sutures, alternate with vertical mattress sutures	—
Leg and thigh	Dermal	3-0 Vicryl simple interrupted sutures	—
	Epidermal	4-0 Monocryl continuous running suture	5-0 Nylon simple interrupted sutures or metal staples
Foot	Epidermal	5-0 Nylon simple interrupted sutures	—

Other studies have suggested that the Insorb staples may be superior to metal staples with respect to inflammation, pain, and cosmetic outcome.[31,32]

TOPICAL TISSUE ADHESIVES

- *2-Octylcyanoacrylate (Dermabond).* Tissue adhesive provides an excellent, strong, and flexible method of approximating wound edges. Compared with sutures, staples, and tapes, adhesives provide faster closure[12] and are essentially equivalent to the other methods of closure in terms of cosmetic outcome,[33] infection rate,[34] and dehiscence rate. Adhesives can be used on most parts of the body and have been employed to close wounds ranging from 0.5 to 50 cm in length. Advantages of tissue adhesives include reduced cost, ease of application, absence of needles and suture removal, and higher rate of patient satisfaction;[35] the major disadvantage is lack of strength. Tissue adhesives should not be applied to tissues within wounds; they should be applied to intact skin at wound edge to hold the injured surfaces together. In addition, these products should not be used for wounds in mucous membranes,[2] contaminated wounds, deep wounds, or wounds under tension.[26,36] Adhesives are particularly useful in superficial wounds or wounds in which the deep dermis has been closed with sutures. The avoidance of postoperative suture removal is beneficial, particularly in the pediatric population.[37] Dermabond used over sutures at the time of surgery[7] provides extra support,[6,38] creates an impermeable suture line, decreases the need for postoperative care, and may reduce redness on the suture line.

TAPES

- *Steri-Strips.* Modern cutaneous tapes have an important roll in wound closure and have certain advantages over sutures and staples. Closure with microporous tape produces far more resistance to infection than other closure techniques.[6] Tapes maintain the integrity of the epidermis, resulting in less tension to the wound.[2] Linear wounds in areas with little tension are easily approximated with tape alone, whereas wounds in areas where the skin is more taut generally require that tape skin closure be supplemented with dermal sutures. In addition, tape will not adhere to mobile areas under tension or moist areas. Retention of sutures in skin wounds beyond a few days may result in slower development of tensile strength than if sutures are removed earlier. Thus, some surgeons prefer to replace cutaneous sutures with tape at 3 to 6 days,[6] and some surgeons prefer to use tape in conjunction with liquid adhesive (Mastisol).[2] If used over sutures at the time of surgery, wound closure tape can relieve tension at the wound edges, provide a partially closed environment, improve the aesthetics of the wound, and reduce the often tedious wound management for which the patient is responsible.[2] Wound edge approximation is less precise with tape alone than with sutures. Wound edema can lead to blistering at the tape margins and to eversion of taped wound edges.

SUMMARY

Numerous options for skin closure have become available in the last 30 years. It is paramount to choose a method tailored to each patient and wound. With excellent technical execution, several methods of closure can achieve similar, high quality results. A full understanding of the biomechanical properties of suture material allows wound closure decisions to be made based on sound scientific knowledge.

ACKNOWLEDGMENTS

Our thanks to Victor Gottlieb MD, Rama P. Mukherjee MD, FRCS, and Alison Wing for their great support and critique.

REFERENCES

1. Van Winkle W Jr, Hastings JC. Considerations in the choice of suture material for various tissues. Surg Gynecol Obstet 1972;135:113–26.
2. Moy RL, Waldman B, Hein DW. A review of sutures and suturing techniques. J Dermatol Surg Oncol 1992;18:785–95.
3. Meyer RD, Antonini CJ. A review of sutures materials, part II. In: Compendium of CME in dentistry. Jamesburg Dental Learning Systems Co.; 1989. p. 360–8.
4. Ammirati CT. Advances in wound closure material. In: James WD, editor, Advances in dermatology, 18. St. Louis (MO): Mosby; 2002. p. 313–38.
5. Szarmach RR, Livingston J, Rodeheaver GT, et al. An innovative surgical suture and needle evaluation and selection program. J Long Term Eff Med Implants 2002;12(4):211–29.
6. Hochberg J, Murray GF. Principles of operative surgery. In: Sabiston DC, editor. Textbook of surgery. 15th edition. Philadelphia: WB Saunders; 1992. p. 253–63.
7. Bloom BS, Golberg D. Suture material in cosmetic cutaneous surgery. J Cosmet Laser Ther 2007;9(1):41–5.
8. Trimbos JB. Security of various knots commonly used in surgical practice. Obstet Gynecol 1984;64:274–80.
9. Bennett RG. Selection of wound closure materials. J Am Acad Dermatol 1988;18: 619–37.
10. Moy RL, Lee A, Zalka A. Commonly used suture materials in skin surgery. Am Fam Physician 1991;44:2123–8.
11. Osther PJ, Gjode P, Mortensen BB, et al. Randomized comparison of polyglycolic acid and polyglyconate sutures for abdominal fascial closure after laparotomy in patients with suspected impaired wound healing. Br J Surg 1995;82:1080–2.
12. Pearl M. Choosing abdominal incision and closure techniques. J Reprod Med 2004;49:662–70.
13. Dumitriu S. Textile-based biomaterials for surgical applications. In: Polymeric biomaterials. London: CRC Press; 2002. p. 512.
14. Gabel EA, Jimenez GP, Eaglstein WH, et al. Performance comparison of nylon and an absorbable suture material (polyglactin 910) in the closure of punch biopsy sites. Dermatol Surg 2000;26:750–2.
15. Ford HR, Jones P, Gaines B, et al. Intraoperative handling and wound healing: controlled clinical trial comparing coated Vicryl plus antibacterial suture (coated polyglactin 910 suture with triclosan) with coated vicryl™ suture (coated polyglactin 910 suture). Surg Infect (Larchmt) 2005;6(3):313–21.
16. Outlaw KK, Vela AR, O'Leary JP. Breaking strength and diameter of absorbable sutures after in vivo exposure in the rat. Am Surg 1998;64:348–54.
17. Debus ES, Geiger D, Sailer M, et al. Physical, biological and handling characteristics of surgical suture material: a comparison of four different multifilament absorbable sutures. Eur Surg Res 1997;29(1):52–61.
18. Niessen FB, Spauwen PH, Kon M. The role of suture material in hypertrophic scar formation: Monocryl™ vs Vicryl Rapide™. Ann Plast Surg 1997;39:254–60.
19. Knoop M, Lunstedt B, Thiede A. Maxon™ and PDS™ – evaluation and physical and biological properties of monofilament absorbable suture materials. Langenbecks Arch Chir 1987;371(1):13–28.

20. Murtha AP, Kaplan AL, Oaglia MJ, et al. Evaluation of a novel technique for wound closure using a barbed suture. Plast Reconstr Surg 2006;117(6):1769–80.
21. Reiter D. Methods and materials for wound closure. Otolaryngol Clin North Am 1995;28(5):1069–79.
22. Wu T. Plastic surgery made easy. Aust Fam Physician 2006;35(7):492–6.
23. Hochberg J, Raman M, Cilento E, et al. Development and evaluation of an in vivo mouse model for studying myocutaneous flaps micro-circulation and viability before and after suturing or stapling. Int J Microcirc Clin Exp 1994;14:67–72.
24. Nahas FX, Ferreira LM, Ghelfond C. Does quilting suture prevent seroma in abdominoplasty? Plast Reconstr Surg 2007;119(3):1060–4.
25. Rink AD, Goldschmidt D, Dietrich J, et al. Negative side effects of retention sutures for abdominal wound closure: a prospective randomized study. Eur J Surg 2000;166:932–7.
26. van Rijssel EJ, Trimbos JB, Booster MH. Mechanical performance of square knots and sliding knots in surgery. Am J Obstet Gynecol 1990;162:93–7.
27. Zeplin PH, Schmidt K, Laske M, et al. Comparison of various methods and material for treatment of skin laceration by a 3-dimensional measuring technique in a pig model. Ann Plast Surg 2007;58:566–72.
28. Adams B, Levy R, Rademaker AE, et al. Frequency of use of suturing and repair techniques preferred by dermatologic surgeons. Dermatol Surg 2006;32:682–9.
29. Lubowski D, Hunt D. Abdominal wound closure comparing the proximate stapler with sutures. Aust N Z J Surg 1985;55:405–6.
30. Fernandez AP, Salopek LS, Rodeheaver PF, et al. A revolutionary advance in skin closure compare to current methods. J Long Term Eff Med Implants 2006;16(1):19–27.
31. Tellis VA. Renal transplant incision closure using new absorbable subcuticular staple device. Clin Transplant 2007;21:410–2.
32. Bozkurt MK, Saydam L. The use of cyanoacrylates for wound closure in head and neck surgery. Eur Arch Otorhinolaryngol 2008;265:331–5.
33. Quinn J, Wells G, Sutcliffe T. Tissue adhesive versus suture wound repair at 1 year: randomize clinical trial correlating early, 3-month, and 1-year cosmetic outcome. Ann Emerg Med 1998;32(6):1–9.
34. Quinn J, Maw J, Ramotar K, et al. Octylcyanoacrylate tissue adhesive versus suture wound repair in a contaminated wound model. Surgery 1997;122:69–72.
35. Bowen ML, Selinger M. Episiotomy closure comparing enbucrilate tissue adhesive with conventional sutures. Int J Gynaecol Obstet 2002;78:201–5.
36. Shapiro AJ, Disnmore RC, North JH Jr. Tensile strength of wound closure with cyanoacrylate glue. Am Surg 2001;67:1113–5.
37. Cooper JM, Paige KT. Primary and revision cleft lip repairs using octyl-2-cyanoacrylate. J Craniofac Surg 2006;17(2):340–3.
38. Komatsu F, Mori R, Uchio Y. Optimum suture material and methods to obtain high tensile strength at knots: problems of conventional knots and the reinforcement effect of adhesive agent. J Orthop Sci 2006;11:70–4.

Skin Flaps

Mary Tschoi, MD[a], Erik A. Hoy, BS[b], Mark S. Granick, MD[a],*

KEYWORDS

- Skin flap • Skin transposition • Reconstructive surgery

Open wounds, particularly around the face, often require complicated techniques for optimal closure. The approach to the closure of the complicated wound depends largely on the nature of the wound, including the location and size of the defect, the functional outcome after closure, the medical comorbidities of the patient, neighboring structures, and whether the defect is secondary to a malignancy or trauma. The goals of wound management are optimal aesthetic outcome, preservation of function, and patient satisfaction.

The authors briefly review basic skin closure options and discuss use of skin flaps, particularly of the head and neck region.

HISTORY OF SKIN FLAPS

The earliest documented surgical intervention to rebuild a complicated defect occurred in India in 700 BC. Sushruta published a description of a forehead flap for nasal reconstruction. This information was not available to Western medicine until the late 1700s, when a British surgeon noted the technique still used in India and wrote a brief description in *Gentleman's Quarterly.*

Independently, the Italians developed delayed flaps, tube flaps, and flap transfers by using the upper inner arm skin to reconstruct a nose. This technique was published by Tagliacozzi in the 1500s. In modern medicine, the use of local flaps to repair facial defects began to evolve during the mid-1800s. A variety of flaps were used, but the blood supply and the dynamics of the surgery were not well understood. Harold Gilles popularized tube flaps and flap delays and initiated an interest in reconstructive surgery after World War I.[1]

Local skin flaps, such as those described in this article, were primarily refined in the 1950s in Europe and the United States by the second generation of plastic surgeons. Ian MacGregor[2,3] recognized the importance of an axial blood supply in flap surgery in the 1970s. Plastic surgeons have subsequently redefined cutaneous blood supply.

This article originally appeared in the May 2005 issue of Clinics in Plastic Surgery.

[a] Division of Plastic Surgery, Department of Surgery, New Jersey Medical School-UMDNJ, 90 Bergen Street, Suite 7200, Newark, NJ 07103, USA

[b] New Jersey Medical School-UMDNJ, 185 South Orange Avenue, Newark, NJ 07103, USA

* Corresponding author.

E-mail address: mgranickmd@umdnj.edu (M.S. Granick).

Surg Clin N Am 89 (2009) 643–658

doi:10.1016/j.suc.2009.03.004

surgical.theclinics.com

Countless vascularized flaps have since been developed. The skin flaps discussed in this article are primarily random flaps.[1–3]

PREOPERATIVE PLANNING AND CONSIDERATIONS

For each patient, a medical history encompassing smoking, peripheral vascular disease, atherosclerosis, diabetes mellitus, steroids, and previous surgeries should be elicited, because of the effects of these factors on wound healing and skin perfusion.

In managing the excisional defect, the surgeon must first assess the size and depth of the wound, as well as the nature of any exposed underlying internal anatomy. A defect containing exposed bone, nerves, or blood vessels usually necessitates a more advanced closure than would a less complicated wound.

The quality of the surrounding skin is also of great importance. Skin quality may vary from young, tight, and elastic to aged, dry, and lax. The wrinkled skin of an older patient produces less obvious scarring and offers the opportunity to conceal scars within skin tension lines. Skin that is more oily or heavily pigmented generally yields a less favorable scar. Color match is also of importance in deciding on the flap donor site. The presence of actinic damage, skin diseases, and premalignant satellite lesions should be considered. Finally, location is of major concern. Defects adjacent to critical anatomic structures, such as the eyelids, the nares, the oral commissure, and the external auditory meatus, must be reconstructed so as to avoid distorting the anatomy unique to those areas. Any alteration of these surrounding landmarks may compromise functional and aesthetic results. Previous surgical incisions and traumatic scars should also be assessed before the closure of the defect is designed.

Well-planned and -executed reconstruction of facial defects is particularly important because of the visibility of the result and the potential for functional deficits. However, the principles presented here may be applied to the management of all complicated wounds.

In the repair of facial tumor defects, the most important consideration is the management of the tumor. Incompletely excised tumor should not be covered by a flap. Skin adjacent to a tumor resection margin should not be turned over to line the nasal cavity or any other site where it will be difficult to examine. In patients who have a history of multiple or recurrent skin cancers, a strategy must be developed to allow for serial repairs. No bridges should be burned along the way. When planning a reconstruction, one must protect function first, then consider the cosmetic issues. It is crucial to discuss options with patients so that they can offer any biases that must be respected. A good-looking static repair that compromises dynamic function is unacceptable. The anatomic boundaries of the face are the allies of a good plastic surgeon. They must be respected and will be helpful in camouflaging scars.

Many defects can be treated with primary closure, secondary healing, or skin grafts. However, if, after careful assessment of the lesion, defect, and patient, the surgeon determines that the patient needs a flap for closure, he or she can apply techniques that produce the optimal aesthetic outcome.

TUMOR RESECTION

The paramount consideration in tumor excision should be the complete removal of the tumor. Although the surgeon should have a number of reconstructive options in mind, the planned reconstruction should not dictate the extent of tumor excision. The surgeon must remain open to alternative reconstructive techniques. If the defect obtained in excising the tumor cannot reasonably be reconstructed at the time of the operation, the wound should be dressed and the reconstruction reconsidered and delayed, or the patient should be referred to another surgeon specializing in these repairs. This option is clearly preferable to a suboptimal reconstruction.

BASIC SKIN CLOSURE TECHNIQUES

Undermining is performed to mobilize the tissue in areas surrounding the defect and to facilitate the draping of skin over the wound. The use of undermining allows the surgeon to move some portions of the wound and not others to avoid the distortion of nearby anatomy, such as the nasolabial fold or the oral commissure. However, because tight closures make for unsightly scars, alternatives should be considered before undermining the edges of a gaping or complicated wound. Undermining can destroy some of the options for flap repair. The reconstruction should be well planned before any undermining. In addition, the surgeon can use closure of the defect in layers to avoid any tension at the wound closure site that might result in dehiscence, wound healing problems, or widened scars.

When using elliptic skin excisions, one should make the long axis four times greater in length than the smaller axis. When an ellipse is made too short or one side of the ellipse is of unequal length, the skin may bunch at one end of the closure. This effect is known as a dog ear. In any wound, whether its sides are of equal or unequal length, the ends of the defect should be closed first to avoid unnecessary dog ears. Any redundancies can be dealt with in the middle of the wound during closure. Irregularities or pleats in the midportion of the wound generally resolve over time. Excising dog ears when they occur is simple. This excision is accomplished by extending the elliptic excision or by cutting the corner of the excision into a Burow's triangle. Alternatively, placing a small right angle or 45° bend in the affected end of the wound closure can produce a satisfactory result. Finally, a V-shaped excision of the lateral ellipse can be used, resulting in an M-plasty closure.

RECONSTRUCTIVE OPTIONS

The final outcome in any closure depends on the proper assessment of the defect and the selection of an appropriate closure technique. Primary closure involving direct approximation of the wound edges is a first option. An intermediate closure consists of approximation and closure of deeper tissue levels before final skin closure. Complex closure entails approximation and adjustment of the wound edges by means of undermining, the excision of any dog ears, or trimming of wound edges before closure. Finally, the options of skin grafting, allografting, and flap repair must be considered.

When a wound cannot be closed primarily, the options are as follows: secondary wound healing, skin grafting (discussed elsewhere), or local tissue transposition. Healing by secondary intention consists of two phenomena. The major means of size reduction of the defect is wound contracture, accompanied by re-epithelization to a lesser extent. Wound contracture may result in distortion of nearby mobile anatomic features, such as the oral commissure or the epicanthi. The contraction of scar tissue alters the orientation of the surrounding normal anatomy, which may result in an unacceptable cosmetic outcome and, more importantly, in poor function.

Healing by secondary intention is a viable option in fixed areas away from important anatomy, such as the middle of the forehead, the cheek, or the neck. In areas adjacent to important, easily deformable anatomic structures, transposition flaps are often a better wound closure approach.[4,5]

SKIN FLAP COVERAGE

Local skin flaps offer several advantages. Well-designed flaps borrow skin from areas of relative excess and transpose it to fill a defect. The skin provided is a close match in both color and texture, the donor site can be closed directly, and scar contracture is minimal. However, these flaps require experience and planning. Preliminarily drawing two or three flap design options for the defect may provide the surgeon with the best visualization of the optimal choice of flap for the particular area and defect. The choice of flap depends on the location and size of the defect, the quality of the surrounding skin, and the location of adjacent excess tissue. One should anticipate the appearance of the donor site scar and, when possible, plan to leave the scar in a natural crease line (eg, the nasolabial fold). When one raises the flap and moves it into the defect, key sutures should be applied and the overall flap position should be evaluated. If there is distortion of adjacent structures, one should reposition the key sutures and re-evaluate again for optimal position and least degree of tension. In addition, once the flap is in place and tacked down with temporary key sutures, it should be assessed for adequate perfusion. Further adjustments may be necessary. Closing the donor site first will relieve tension at the inset location. For example, closure of the Y lower limb in a V-Y flap helps push the flap to the inset position, and suturing on the bias further helps advance the flap into its recipient position. Once the final position of the flap is determined, it can be inset using the basic techniques already mentioned.

FLAP CLASSIFICATION

Flaps were first classified as random or axial by McGregor and Morgan[3] in 1973. Random flaps had no specific vascular supply. Axial flaps had an arterial and venous blood supply in the long axis of the flap. Further contributions to the classification of flaps were made by Daniel and Williams,[6] Webster,[7] Kunert,[8] and Cormack and Lamberty.[9] A random cutaneous flap's blood supply is derived from the dermal-subdermal plexuses of blood vessels, which originate from direct cutaneous, fasciocutaneous, or musculocutaneous vessels. One example is the rhomboid flap. The arterial, axial, and direct cutaneous flaps are based on septocutaneous arteries. These septocutaneous arteries come either from segmental or muscular vessels, pass through the fascia between muscles, and provide blood supply to the fascia and skin. They also give off branches to the muscle. The cutaneous portion of the septocutaneous arteries runs parallel to the skin surface and has venous comitantes running along with the artery above the muscle. An example is a forehead flap. In summary, survival of the skin flap is dependent on the vascular anatomy incorporated in the flap.[10–12]

TRANSPOSITION FLAPS

Local transposition flaps involve the movement of adjacent skin from an area of excess to the area of deficiency. These flaps involve the transfer of the flap through an arc of rotation on a pivot point in a linear axis. Regional tissue laxity and mobility are of greater importance than the precise angular/geometric measurements. In addition, the flap should be designed to fit the defect with minimal tension at the closure line, to avoid distorting the neighboring structures, and to have an adequate base to perfuse the undermined, elevated flap. The rule of thumb is that the random pattern transposition flaps should not have a linear axis longer than three times the width of the flap. Rhomboid flaps, Z-plasties, and W-plasties are variations on the transposition flap. They involve the transposition of a random skin and subcutaneous tissue flap into an adjoining defect. These flaps are designed so that the donor scar is well camouflaged. They must be meticulously designed according to the specific requirements of the reconstruction. However, transposition flaps are quick and easy for the experienced surgeon and are versatile solutions to many coverage problems. Particular areas well-suited to transposition flaps include the glabela, temple region, scalp, and lower third of the nose. Smokers and other patients with vascular compromise are at risk for flap necrosis.[13,14]

Banner Flap

The banner flap (**Fig. 1**)[15] is a transposition flap designed as a pendant of skin tangential to the edge of a round defect. The flap is elevated, and the donor site closed. The flap edges are then trimmed to fit the defect better, and the flap is inset.

The bilobed flap (**Fig. 2**)[16–20] is a variant of the banner flap in which two adjacent segments are raised, one smaller than the other. The two flaps are oriented perpendicularly to each other. The smaller flap (usually half the diameter of the larger flap) is used to fill the larger donor site, and the small donor site is closed primarily. The original defect is then closed by means of the larger of the two lobes. The final result is the 180° rotation of excess tissue to fill the skin deficit. Bilobed flaps are most commonly used in the closure of nasal defects, particularly in the lower third, and they are a means to transfer excess adjacent skin into the area of deficiency. Defects that cannot be covered using a single transposition flap because of tension can be closed by this method. One must be aware that these curvilinear incisions will not necessarily fall into pre-existing skin folds or wrinkles.

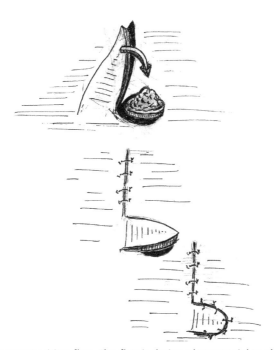

Fig. 1. The banner transposition flap. The flap is designed tangential to the defect and the donor site closed primarily.

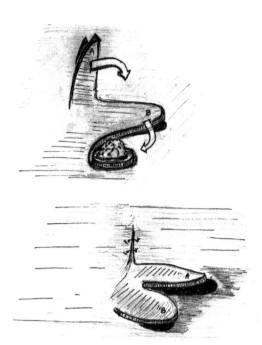

Fig. 2. The bilobed transposition flap. The primary donor flap is designed tangential to the defect, and the secondary flap is designed to be smaller and more elliptic to allow for primary closure of the secondary donor site.

Rhomboid Flap

Rhomboid flaps (**Fig. 3**)[21–25] are rhomboid-shaped skin flaps transposed into like-shaped defects leaving an angulated donor site, which can then be closed primarily. A corner of the rhombus is extended at a length equal to one of the short diagonals. This new limb is joined by another at a 60° angle. Because all rhomboids possess four corners that can be extended, any rhomboid defect is amenable to any of eight possible rhomboid flaps. The end result is a scar of geometric appearance, which is best when hidden in the natural crease lines of the skin. Although the customary angles are 60° and 120°, variations of the rhomboid flap using 30° and 150° angles are possible. These variations allow for coverage of rhomboid defects with unequal sides. Because this approach involves more meticulous planning, it is sometimes simpler to begin by converting the defect into a rhombus of 60° and 120° angles. The area of maximum tension is at the closure point of the donor site flap. The vector of maximum tension has been determined to be 20° to the short diagonal of the rhomboid defect. Every rhomboid defect has eight potential flaps for closure, and it is up to the surgeons to decide which donor site is optimal.

When a larger wound needs to be closed, the circular defect can be converted into a hexagon and closed with three rhomboid flaps. This procedure is even more complicated to plan, and it leaves a stellate-shaped scar. The scar is difficult to merge into natural crease lines and is consequently noticeable as a geometric scar. This technique should be used with caution.

Z-plasty

The Z-plasty (**Fig. 4**) is a double transposition flap that is often an appropriate option in scar revision or in the release of scar contractions. These flaps are well suited to the

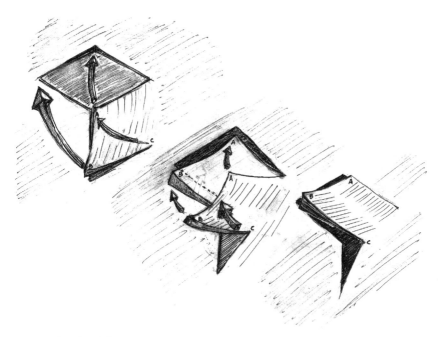

Fig. 3. The rhomboid flap.

correction of skin webs and the disruption of circumferential scars or constricting bands. Furthermore, the Z-plasty elongates the operated tissues.

The Z-plasty entails the exchange of two adjacent triangular flaps. The incision consists of a central limb and two limbs oriented to resemble a Z. All limbs are the same length to facilitate closure. The length of the central limb dictates the absolute gain in length after Z-plasty, whereas the angles chosen determine the percentage of length increase. The typical Z-plasty has 60° angles, resulting in a gain in length of 70% relative to the central limb. The angles may range from 30° to 90°, providing gains in length of 25% and 120%, respectively.[4] However, these gains are theoretic. Smaller gains are seen in practice because of restrictive skin factors. Because the Z-plasty relies on healthy adjacent skin, it is usually a poor choice for the correction of burn scar contractures. However, the gain in length granted by the Z-plasty is well suited to other scar contractures, and the changed axis of the final scar often provides a more desirable aesthetic result in facial scar revision.

When laying out the Z-plasty, one should plot the final position of the central limb first. This final position is perpendicular to the original central limb incision and should be oriented parallel to the skin lines. Consecutive Z-plasties result in further transposition of skin and obliteration of straight-line scars. Multiple Z-plasties produce transverse shortening and lateral tension on the wound.

W-plasty

The W-plasty is similar to a Z-plasty in its ability to break up a linear scar. A defect is created by removing a scar or lesion in a precise, premarked zigzag pattern that creates multiple small triangular flaps. The multiple triangular flaps are interposed among one another. The base of each triangle is aligned with the vertex of the one opposite. Unlike the Z-plasty, the W-plasty does not confer any gain in length on

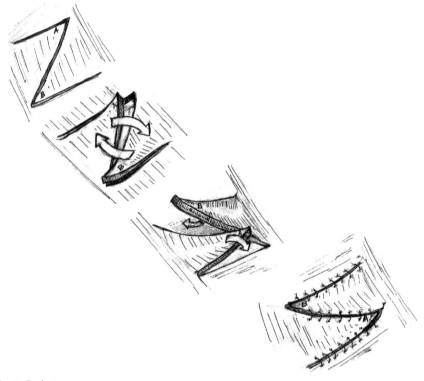

Fig. 4. Z-plasty.

the contracted scar line. As the ends of the scar are approached, the triangles should decrease in size, and the limbs of the triangles should decrease as well.

ROTATION FLAPS

Rotation flaps (**Fig. 5**)[4,13,26] are semicircular flaps raised in a subdermal plane and rotated from the donor bed around a pivot point adjacent to the defect. The defect site is visualized as a triangle with its base as the shortest side. After the flap is rotated into the defect, the donor site is closed primarily, yielding an arcuate scar. Considerable tension may be present in this flap and needs to be recognized. The line of maximal tension is directly opposite the pivot point and adjacent to the defect. Excessive tension along this line may result in ischemia and subsequent necrosis of the flap. Rotation flaps require considerable planning, and little gain is realized relative to the

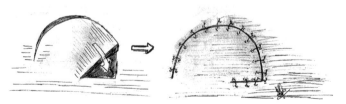

Fig. 5. Rotation flap.

size of the flap. In some cases, the donor site cannot be closed primarily and may require a skin graft. However, depending on the location of the defect, rotation flaps may be preferable to transposition or advancement flaps.

A problem with rotational flaps is the unequal length between the edge of the flap and the entire edge of the primary and secondary defects. To correct this mismatch in length, one can use the Burow's triangle technique, a cutback incision, advancement of the flap while rotating it, or suture on the bias to stretch the flap forward. The rule of thumb is that the length of the flap should be four times the width of the base of the defect. In addition, the ideal defect for repair has a height to width ratio of two to one. The blood supply is usually random, but if the surgeon designs the position of the base of the flap, it can be axial.

ADVANCEMENT FLAPS

Advancement flaps involve raising a skin paddle in a subdermal plane and moving its leading edge into the defect. The movement of the flap is longitudinal rather than rotational and is directly over the defect. Complete undermining of the flap is very important. Burow's triangles are often excised at the base of the flap to remove dog ears as the flap advances relative to the surrounding skin. These flaps have limited coverage potential and utility. The single-pedicle advancement flap is the basic flap. The ratio of defect length to flap length is one to three. Bilateral advancement flaps may be used if a single flap does not provide adequate tension-free closure of the defect.[4,13,14]

V-Y Plasty

V-Y plasty (**Fig. 6**)[27,28] is a variation of the advancement flap. In a V-Y plasty, the skin flap is not elevated and remains attached to the underlying subcutaneous tissues. A V-shaped flap is designed adjacent to the defect. The surrounding skin is elevated, and the V-shaped tissue is advanced into the wound. The donor site is closed primarily, yielding a Y-shaped closure. It may be necessary to trim the triangular edges of the leading flap to fit into the defect. This technique is particularly well suited to elongating the nasal columella and correcting the whistle deformity of the lip. The V-Y flap is one of the most versatile skin flaps and is widely used in all areas of the face.

Island Flap

Island flaps, as their name implies, involve the transposition of an island of skin that is raised on its blood supply. The skin island is moved into the defect, and the donor site is closed primarily. Often, this involves tunneling the flap under adjacent skin on its vascular pedicle. The flap island should be approximately the size of the defect to

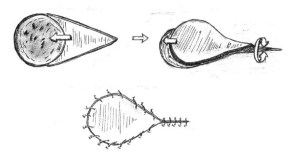

Fig. 6. V-Y advancement flap.

be covered. In areas such as the eyebrow, the island flap provides a supply of like tissue without permitting the distortion of normal anatomy. A circular island flap may pin-cushion. This complication can be avoided with proper planning.[4,13,14]

T-plasty

T-plasty is an advancement technique that converts a triangular or circular defect into an inverted-T scar. It is essentially a bilateral advancement flap and works well in the central forehead, above the eyebrows, and on the upper lip just above the vermilion. Care must be taken, because the vertical limb of the T can be noticeable in some areas.[13]

CLINICAL SCENARIOS

Many options are available for closing defects of the face and other areas of the body; the authors outline only a few of them here. The reconstruction of each defect must be individualized to attain the optimal aesthetic outcome. In each of the following clinical cases, multiple skin flap options are discussed for each defect. These are, of course, not the only options, and the selected reconstruction is not the only good choice. The principles of selecting an appropriate repair are the same in each case.

Fig. 7A depicts a 65-year-old woman who underwent excision of basal cell carcinoma and now has a 2.5-cm defect in the side of her nose. Aesthetic reconstruction of nasal deficits is a common problem posed to the reconstructive surgeon by the high

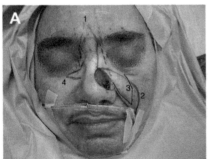
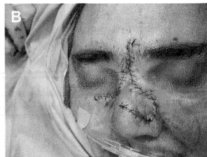
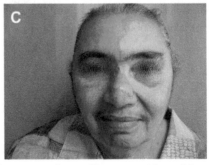

Fig. 7. (*A*) A 65-year-old woman who underwent excision of basal cell carcinoma with a 2.5-cm defect in the side of the nose. (1) Transposition glabelar flap. (2) Advancement flap following the nasolabial groove medially. (3) Nasolabial flap. (4) Bilobed glabelar flap. (*B*) Intraoperative photograph of patient after the bilobed glabelar flap with the donor site closed in a Y-fashion. (*C*) Postoperative photograph of the bilobed glabelar flap.

incidence of nasal skin cancer. Several considerations need to be addressed in the reconstruction of nasal defects: color and texture match, minimization of bulkiness, appreciation of discrete aesthetic units of the nose, skin tension lines and wrinkles, adequacy of tissue, and vascularity.

- The glabelar skin offers an excellent source of tissue for nasal repairs. The transposition glabelar flap provides good skin match and adequate skin to cover this defect, and the glabelar region can be closed primarily with a vertical scar orientation at the donor site that can be easily camouflaged.
- The incision can be made along the nasolabial groove and along the cheek, following natural skin lines, to raise an advancement flap. This flap is advanced medially to cover the defect. The cheek has good skin laxity to close the defect at its base. However, the bulkiness of the cheek relative to the nasal skin may be obvious.
- A nasolabial flap[29] can be elevated in the subcutaneous plane of the cheek and transposed to the defect. In this case, a dog ear needs to be excised at the pivot point superiorly. The cheek has to be undermined beyond the flap to allow for transposition of this flap. The donor site can be closed primarily, with the closure falling along the nasolabial fold. Closure of the donor site would disrupt the eyelid-cheek skin lines.
- A bilobed glabelar flap can be used, as in this case (**Fig. 7**B), to cover the defect. The smaller lobe is transposed to cover the donor defect. The rest of the glabelar region site can be closed primarily in a Y fashion. Good skin color and texture match are seen, with minimal tension and good camouflage of scars (**Fig. 7**C).

Fig. 8A shows a 62-year-old man with a cheek defect after resection of squamous cell carcinoma. The defect is 4.5 cm in size and lies 3.5 cm lateral to the mouth.

- An advancement flap may be designed, based either laterally or inferiorly, to close this defect. Parallel incisions can be made, raised in the subcutaneous plane, and advanced to cover the defect. Good laxity of the skin of the cheek, especially in the elderly, provides sufficient tissue for the repair. Dog ears at the base of the flap can be excised. The inferiorly based advancement flap takes advantage of the laxity of the skin of the neck, and the scar lines fall in the natural skin lines. Hence, the inferiorly based advancement flap is a better option than the laterally based one.
- A banner flap can also be used to transpose into the defect. However, the scar may not be as easily camouflaged.
- Other options include (1) a cheek rotation flap, (2) a rhomboid flap inferiorly based to take advantage of the lax skin of the neck, and (3) a V-Y advancement flap based laterally (**Figs. 8**B and **8**C).[30,31]

In the patient shown in **Fig. 9**A, the defect is centrally located in the dorsum of the nose. Several good options are available for its reconstruction.

- A superiorly based V-Y advancement flap may be used.
- A rotation glabelar flap may be used and a backcut designed to close the donor site pivot point in a Y configuration (**Fig. 9**B).[32]
- A rhomboid flap would not be the ideal design, because the nasal skin is not as mobile and may distort the medial canthus and create a web or ectropion. It is important that the design of the flap in this patient lie within the wrinkles of the face to mask the scar and not distort the eyebrows and eyes.

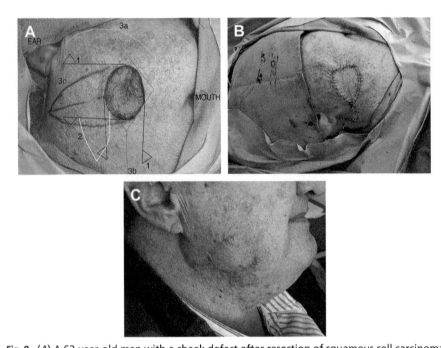

Fig. 8. (*A*) A 62-year-old man with a cheek defect after resection of squamous cell carcinoma 4.5 cm in size. (1) Advancement flap based laterally or inferiorly with excision of Burow's triangles. (2) Banner flap. (3a) Cheek rotation flap. (3b) Rhomboid flap. (3c) V-Y advancement flap. (*B*) Intraoperative photograph of patient after the V-Y advancement flap of the cheek defect. (*C*) Postoperative photograph of patient after the V-Y advancement flap of the cheek defect.

A banner flap may also be designed, using the tissue available from the side wall of the nose and primary closure of the donor site.

Fig. 10A shows an 85-year-old woman after resection of basal cell carcinoma from her upper lip, creating a 1.5-cm circular defect. This defect lies just above the vermilion and medial to the nasolabial fold and is close to the alar base, philtrum, and cupid's bow.

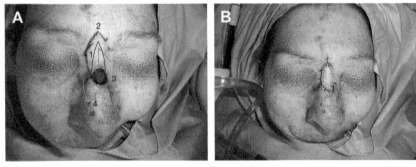

Fig. 9. (*A*) Patient with a dorsal nose defect. (1) Superiorly based V-Y advancement flap. (2) Rotation glabelar flap and a backcut to close the donor site. (3) Rhomboid flap. (4) Banner flap. (*B*) Intraoperative photograph of rotation glabelar flap with a backcut to close the donor site in a Y-fashion.

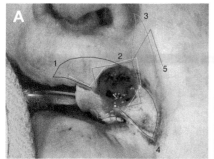
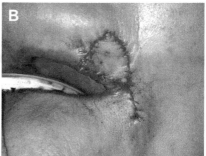
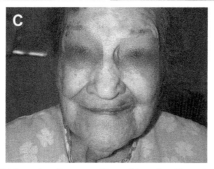

Fig. 10. (*A*) An 85-year-old female after resection of basal cell carcinoma from the upper lip with a 1.5-cm defect resulting. (1) Bilateral V-Y advancement flap. (2) A-T advancement flap. (3) Nasolabial flap. (4) Single V-Y advancement along the nasolabial fold and vermilion border. (5) Rhomboid flap would distort the nasolabial fold to a greater degree than the other flaps mentioned. (*B*) Intraoperative photograph of V-Y advancement flap in the upper lip. (*C*) Postoperative photograph of V-Y advancement flap.

A bilateral V-Y advancement flap may be used to close the defect with adequate undermining. Excellent laxity of the skin and natural skin folds and wrinkles are present and may be used to the surgeon's advantage. However, the medial V-Y flap may distort the cupid's bow.

An A-T advancement flap may also be used, by taking a triangular wedge out superiorly from the defect and undermining on both sides to close the defect.

A nasolabial flap may be used by raising the flap along the nasolabial fold.

A single V-Y advancement flap was designed, following the vermilion border and the nasolabial fold to advance medially into the defect (**Figs. 10**B and **10**C).[33]

A rhomboid flap, in this case, would distort the nasolabial fold and would not mask the scar as well.

FOLLOW-UP CARE

Follow-up care is an important aspect of the treatment of any surgical wound. Suture removal is timed to prevent suture cross marks and epithelial cysts. Patients need to be advised as to the proper management of new scars and monitored to ensure that the healing process is progressing normally. As in the treatment of any condition, follow-up and continuity of care are vital aspects of good medical practice. Skin flaps take 3 to 6 months to mature. They tend to look puffy and distorted at first but will settle down and improve over time. Patients need to be reassured.

EARLY COMPLICATIONS OF FLAP RECONSTRUCTION

The possible complications after flap reconstruction vary in severity and require distinct approaches depending on their type. Fortunately, most of the complications are preventable as well as amenable to treatment. The most common early complications after skin flap reconstruction surgery are infection, hematoma, seroma, and wound dehiscence.

The complication of flap necrosis is more serious and is usually due to a design flaw or an error in execution of the reconstruction. These errors include the use of too small a flap for a given defect, damage to the flap's blood supply, extension of the flap beyond its blood supply, or closure of the defect in such a way that it is subject to too much tension. Flap necrosis may usually be avoided by means of more precise flap design and avoidance of undue tension on wound closure. Treatment of distal necrosis is conservative and may include allowing certain areas to heal by secondary intention or subsequent surgical revision of the area. However, in areas where the flap was placed to prevent a deforming scar contracture, such as the eyelid, a new reconstruction should be performed as soon as the wound condition permits.

LATE COMPLICATIONS OF FLAP RECONSTRUCTION

These complications are avoided for the most part by means of experience and careful planning of the flap reconstruction. Unfavorable scarring is a complication that occurs when scars are placed outside of the direction of the skin tension lines. Scars that lie in the wrong direction may be revised with a Z-plasty or a W-plasty. Pin-cushioning (trap door deformity) of the flap is another complication that arises from a curvilinear scar. Correction of the pin-cushion deformity should not be performed until the scar matures. Options for correction include excision of the old scar, defatting of the flap, and closure with Z-plasties or a W-plasty.

Hypertrophic scars are uncommon on the face. However, keloids can be a major concern. Any patient with a personal or family history of keloids or a personal history of hypertrophic scars must be warned about the risk of developing additional keloids or hypertrophic scars. Once a keloid forms, many treatment options are available, most of which are only partially effective in minimizing the scar. Pressure, topical silicone, steroid injections, and massage are the standard treatments, although re-excision in conjunction with intralesional steroids and postoperative radiation may also be considered for unresponsive lesions.

OUTCOME AND PROGNOSIS

When local flaps are insufficient to cover a wound properly, distant tissue may be imported using techniques such as skin grafting, pedicled flaps, axial flaps, fasciocutaneous flaps, myocutaneous flaps, and free flaps. If the removal of sutures that are too tight or the correction of a hematoma delays the repair, this is a small price to pay for the avoidance of flap necrosis and a better end-result. The primary goal in tumor surgery is adequate treatment of the tumor. Only after that treatment may a definitive reconstruction be undertaken. The reconstruction must preserve function and provide the best possible cosmetic result.

ACKNOWLEDGMENTS

Special thanks to Dr. Gordon Kaplan, Plastic Surgery Resident, UMDNJ/New Jersey Medical School, for his artistic contribution to this manuscript and to Michelle Granick for providing her expertise with the digital photographs.

REFERENCES

1. Converse JM. Introduction to plastic surgery. In: Converse JM, editor. 2nd edition, Reconstructive plastic surgery, Vol. 1. Philadelphia: WB Saunders; 1977. p. 3–68.
2. McGregor IA. Design of skin flaps. Lancet 1970;2(2):130–3.
3. McGregor IA, Morgan G. Axial and random pattern flaps. Br J Plast Surg 1973;26: 202–13.
4. Place MJ, Herber SC, Hardesty RA. Basic techniques and principles in plastic surgery. In: Grabb and Smith's Plastic Surgery. 5th edition. Boston: Lippincott-Raven; 1997. p. 13–26.
5. Lamberty BGH, Healy C. Flaps: physiology, principles of design, and pitfalls. In: Cohen M, editor, Mastery of plastic and reconstructive surgery, Vol. 1. Boston: Little, Brown and Co.; 1994. p. 56–70.
6. Daniel RK, Williams HB. The free transfer of skin flaps by microvascular anastomoses: an experimental study and a reappraisal. Part I: the vascular supply of the skin. Plast Reconstr Surg 1973;52:16–31.
7. Webster JP. Thoraco-epigastric tubed pedicles. Surg Clin North Am 1937;17:145.
8. Kunert P. Structure and construction: the system of skin flaps. Ann Plast Surg 1991;27:509–16.
9. Cormack GC, Lamberty BGH. A classification of fasciocutaneous flaps according to their patterns of vascularization. Br J Plast Surg 1984;37:80–7.
10. Daniel RK, Kerrigan CL. Principles and physiology of skin flaps. In: McCarthy JG, editor, Plastic surgery, Vol. 1. Philadelphia: WB Saunders; 1990. p. 275–328.
11. Kayser MR, Hodges PL, Surgical flaps. In: Barton Jr FE, editor. Selected readings in plastic surgery. Vol. 8, No. 3. Dallas (TX): Baylor University Medical Center; 1995. p. 1–58
12. Taylor GI. The blood supply of the skin. In: Grabb and Smith's Plastic Surgery. 5th edition. Boston: Lippincott-Raven; 1997. p. 47–60.
13. Baker SR, Swanson NA. Local flaps in facial reconstruction. St. Louis: Mosby; 1995.
14. Jackson IT. Local flaps in head and neck reconstruction. St. Louis: Quality Medical Publishing; 1985.
15. Masson JK, Mendelson BC. The banner flap. Am J Surg 1977;134(3):419–23.
16. Zitelli JA. The bilobed flap for nasal reconstruction. Arch Dermatol 1989;125(7): 957–9.
17. McGregor JC, Soutar DS. A critical assessment of the bilobed flap. Br J Plast Surg 1981;34(2):197–205.
18. Golcman R, Speranzini MB, Golcman B. The bilobed island flap in nasal ala reconstruction. Br J Plast Surg 1998;51(7):493–8.
19. Zimany A. The bi-lobed flap. Facial Plast Surg Clin North Am 1953;11:424–34.
20. Morgan BL, Samiian MR. Advantages of the bilobed flap for closure of small defects of the face. Plast Reconstr Surg 1973;52(1):35–7.
21. Bray DA. Clinical applications of the rhomboid flap. Arch Otolaryngol 1983; 109(1):37–42.
22. Borges AF. The rhombic flap. Plast Reconstr Surg 1981;67(4):458–66.
23. Borges AF. Choosing the correct Limberg flap. Plast Reconstr Surg 1978;62(4): 542–5.
24. Becker FF. Rhomboid flap in facial reconstruction. New concept of tension lines. Arch Otolaryngol 1979;105(10):569–73.
25. Lober CW, Mendelsohn HE, Fenske NA. Rhomboid transposition flaps. Aesthetic Plast Surg 1985;9(2):121–4.

26. Green RK, Angelats J. A full nasal skin rotation flap for closure of soft-tissue defects in the lower one-third of the nose. Plast Reconstr Surg 1996;98(1):163–6.
27. Cronin TD. The V-Y rotational flap for nasal tip defects. Ann Plast Surg 1983;11(4): 282–8.
28. Omidi MS, Granick MS. The versatile V-Y flap for facial reconstruction. Dermatol Surg 2004;30(3):415–20.
29. Zitelli JA. The nasolabial flap as a single-stage procedure. Arch Dermatol 1990; 126(11):1445–8.
30. Schrudde J, Beinhoff U. Reconstruction of the face by means of the angle-rotation flap. Aesthetic Plast Surg 1987;11(1):15–22.
31. Yotsuyanagi T, Yamashita K, Urushidate S, et al. Reconstruction of large nasal defects with a combination of loca flaps based on the aesthetic subunit principle. Plast Reconstr Surg 2001;107(6):1358–62.
32. Rigg BM. The dorsal nasal flap. Plast Reconstr Surg 1973;52(4):361–4.
33. Carvalho LM, Ramos RR, Santos ID, et al. V-Y advancement flap for the reconstruction of partial and full thickness defects of the upper lip. Scand J Plast Reconstr Surg Hand Surg 2002;36(1):28–33.

Management of Acute Wounds

Charles K. Lee, MD[a,b],*, Scott L. Hansen, MD[a,c]

KEYWORDS

- Wounds • Surgical debridement • Skin graft • Wound care
- Management and dressings • Free flaps
- Reconstructive plastic surgery • Wound healing

The acute wound presents a spectrum of issues that prevent its ultimate closure. These issues include host factors, etiology, anatomic location, timing, and surgical techniques to achieve successful wound closure. Basic surgical principles need to be followed to obtain stable, long-term coverage, ultimately restoring form and function. Recent advances in dressings, debridement techniques, and surgical repertoire allow the modern plastic surgeon to address any wound of any complexity. This article discusses these principles that can be applied to any wound.

DEFINITION OF THE ACUTE WOUND

The acute wound is a breakdown of the integrity of the soft tissue envelope surrounding any portion of the body. It is defined by size, depth, and involved anatomic structures. The time course between an acute versus chronic wound is a continuum between 4 and 6 weeks. It is during this time that if an acute wound has not healed spontaneously, it is likely to become a chronic, "problem wound" that requires further intervention.[1] The acute wound can present as simple or complex, depending on its location, size, involved anatomic structures, and bioburden. The foundation for closure of an acute wound lies in an adequate surgical debridement and a systematic approach to options for closure.

MECHANISM/ETIOLOGY

The acute wound is created by the violation of the skin and subcutaneous tissue integrity through multiple mechanisms. These mechanisms include penetrating or blunt trauma as well as various environmental exposures, such as chemical substances,

This article Originally appeared in the October 2007 issue of *Clinics in Plastic Surgery*.

[a] University of California, San Francisco, 350 Parnassus, Suite 509, San Francisco, CA 94117, USA
[b] St. Mary's Medical Center, San Francisco, 2250 Hayes Street, Suite 508, San Francisco, CA 94117, USA
[c] San Francisco General Hospital, Ward 3A, Box 0807, San Francisco, CA 94143, USA
* Corresponding author. St. Mary's Medical Center, San Francisco, 2250 Hayes Street, Suite 508, San Francisco, CA 94117.
E-mail address: leeplasticsurgery@gmail.com (C.K. Lee).

extremes of temperature, prolonged or excessive pressure, and radiation. Disruption of the continuity of the skin from any of these mechanisms allows entry of organisms that can lead to local or systemic infection.

Traumatic Injuries

Traumatic injuries can be subdivided into blunt or penetrating trauma. Blunt trauma can result in a large area of tissue destruction, the extent of which is not always obvious. Crush, degloving, and avulsion injuries fall into a similar category; it is difficult to determine the extent of tissue viability on initial examination. In these situations, the mechanism of injury translates into a larger anatomic zone based on direct tissue destruction and microvascular injury. These types of injuries require thorough exploration and subsequent vigilance to identify the zones of injury.

The "zone of injury" is divided into three areas: the zone of necrosis (obviously necrotic tissue), the zone of stasis (adjacent to the zone of necrosis and extremely vulnerable to necrosis), and the zone of hyperemia (outside the zone of stasis with viable tissue.[2] Determining these zones clinically in an acute, complex wound is not a simple task; however, with aggressive debridement of nonviable tissue, bacteriologic control, and fluid resuscitation, the zones of stasis and hyperemia can be maintained and delineated.

Penetrating trauma results in the destruction of soft tissues with variable amounts of underlying tendon, nerve, bone, or vascular disruption (**Figs. 1–3**). Gunshot injuries represent a specific type of penetrating injury. Depending on the caliber of the weapon, wounds may involve minimal soft tissue loss with underlying tissue destruction to complete destruction of soft tissues in addition to underlying muscle, bone, tendon, nerve, and blood vessels. Damage is caused by several mechanisms: laceration and crush, shock waves, and cavitation. These acute wounds present a challenge for the tissue destruction as well as because of the violation of functional structures of the body.

Other acute traumatic wounds occur from human and animal bites. These acute wounds need attention for their potential serious morbidity from infection. Often, human bite wounds are underestimated because of their early benign appearance. Late presentation with serious infection through tissue planes call for "overestimation" of the problem on initial presentation. Bacteria isolated from human bite wounds are numerous. Commonly isolated aerobic organisms include α- and β-hemolytic streptococci, *Staphylococcus aureus*, *Staphylococcus epidermis*, *Corynebacterium* spp., and *Eikenella corrodens*. Commonly isolated anaerobic organisms include *Peptostreptococcus* spp., *Bacteroides* (*fragilis* and *nonfragilis* spp.), *Fusobacterium*, *Veillonella*, *Prevotella*, *Porphyromonas*, and *Clostridium*.

Dog and cat bites are common animal bites. Dog bites have the potential to cause significant wounds secondary to crush and avulsion. An adult dog can exert 200 pounds per square inch (psi) of pressure, with some larger dogs able to exert

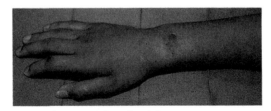

Fig. 1. Entry wound for gunshot wound to distal forearm.

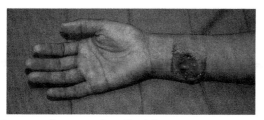

Fig. 2. Exit wound from gunshot wound to distal forearm.

450 psi.[3] The cat bite, although less powerful than a dog, can be equally dangerous from their pointed teeth that allow inoculation of deep tissues. Common bacteria involved in dog bites include *Staphylococcus*, *Streptococcus*, *Eikenella*, *Pasteurella*, *Proteus*, and *Klebsiella*.[4] Common bacteria involved in cat bites include *Pasteurella*, *Actinomyces*, *Propionibacterium*, *Bacteroides*, *Fusobacterium*, and *Clostridium*.

Envenomation

Toxins may be delivered by insect or reptile bites, which result in acute wounds. The venomous exposure can act on the tissues locally or systemically as a neurotoxin. The most common insect bite associated with severe tissue necrosis is that of the brown recluse spider (*Loxosceles reclusa*). The toxins from the brown recluse spider cause painful, necrotic, and slow-healing wounds. The mechanism for this skin necrosis is not entirely understood, but it is believed to be dependent on the victim's neutrophil function. The Loxosceles venom acts as an endothelial cell agonist, stimulating an inflammatory response, which eventually leads to dysregulated neutrophil function. The black widow spider (*Latrodectus* spp.) can produce severe skin lesions that may lead to an acute wound. Local envenomation begins with pain and pruritis that progresses to vesiculation with violaceous necrosis, surrounding erythema, and ulcer formation. The venom from the black widow spider is called α-latrotoxin and is a potent neurotoxin.

The venom from a snake bite contains many toxic proteins and enzymes that have potentially harmful consequences. The components of the toxins are many and include procoagulants, anticoagulants, hyaluronidases, RNases, DNases, postsynaptic toxins, and presynaptic toxins. Other animals that produce toxins include scorpions, lizards, and marine animals. The acute wounds vary in size and complexity depending on the volume and type of toxin.

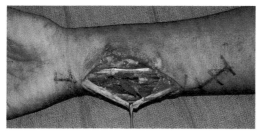

Fig. 3. Exploration of the wound reveals significant neurovascular, muscle, and tendon injury.

Exposure to Chemical Substances

Many substances can disrupt the integrity of the skin. Injuries that are seen commonly by physicians are those that are caused by environmental chemicals (alkali or acidic solutions) or those that may occur iatrogenically as a complication of intravenous (IV) fluid administration. These are considered chemical burns and are covered in detail elsewhere in this issue in the article on burns.

IV fluid that extravasates into the peripheral tissues during an infusion is a common cause of an acute wound (**Figs. 4** and **5**). IV fluid extravasation is defined as leakage of injectable fluids out of the vein into the interstitial space. This problem may be the result of a displacement of the IV line or may result from increased vascular permeability. Depending on the solution being injected, surrounding tissue may be injured to varying degrees. The most common substances that extravasate are cationic solutions (eg, potassium ion, calcium ion, bicarbonate), osmotically active chemicals (eg, total parenteral nutrition or hypertonic dextrose solutions), antibiotics, and cytotoxic drugs. Extravasation causes tissue necrosis from chemical toxicity, osmotic toxicity, or the effects of pressure in a closed environment. In most instances, the tissue necrosis is underestimated. Following extravasation, edema, erythema, and induration usually are present with variable amounts of necrotic tissue, the extent of which is not readily apparent.

Paint gun injection (**Fig. 6**) injuries pose another threat to soft tissue integrity. High-powered paint guns deliver chemicals through a small nozzle at 2000 to 10,000 psi. These paint guns can cause devastating injuries, most commonly to the hand through a single digit. Significant injury results from vascular compression, chemical inflammation, and secondary infection. Fuel and paint injections have the highest morbidity because the solvents that are used to counteract and remove these products also are toxic.

Temperature

Skin that is exposed to extremes of temperature is at risk for injury, including hyper- and hypothermic injuries (hyperthermic injuries are covered elsewhere in this issue). Hypothermic injuries can result in severe frostbite, the severity of which is related to the duration of exposure and to the temperature gradient at the skin surface.[4–6] It has been shown experimentally that the tensile strength of a healing wound decreases by 20% in a cold (12°C) environment.

Frostbite occurs by the formation of ice crystals in the intracellular and extracellular space. During the cooling process, the extracellular ice crystals form, and osmotic pressure increases, drawing water out of the cells. This leads to intracellular dehydration with an increase in intracellular electrolytes, proteins, and enzymes that lead to cell death. Additionally, there is vascular endothelial damage leading to intravascular thrombosis and reduced blood flow. Arterio-venous shunting occurs at the capillary level, and end-organ tissue damage is compounded. During the warming process, there is an influx of fluid back into the cells causing intracellular swelling. The warming

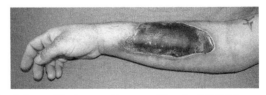

Fig. 4. Extravasation injury with demarcation, resulting in full-thickness skin loss.

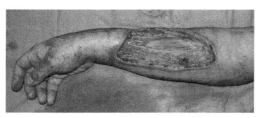

Fig. 5. After debridement of the eschar.

process also allows reflow, vasodilation, and reactive hyperemia to occur, leading to increased inflammatory mediators, causing further cell death.

Severe frostbite injuries have occurred through natural and iatrogenic injuries and are becoming more common in the postoperative setting with cooling devices (**Fig. 7**).[5]

Surgery

Tissue injury may occur from elective or emergency surgical procedures creating an acute wound. Postsurgical wounds may become complicated because of a disruption or an injury to the local or regional blood supply. Along with proper atraumatic tissue handling and selective blood vessel cauterization, skin approximation must not be placed under excessive tension to avoid skin and soft tissue necrosis. Skin necrosis from vascular disruption or excessive tension at closure may lead to poor wound healing and eventually lead to an acute open wound.

When a surgical procedure involves elevation of skin and subcutaneous tissue with disruption of deep fascial and muscle vascular connections, the survival of the subcutaneous tissue and skin depend on the blood supply in the dermal–subdermal plexus. Cutaneous flap survival is limited by the disruption of this plexus, which can lead to tissue necrosis and subsequent bacterial infection.

Oncologic resection also creates an acute, iatrogenic wound, which often requires immediate reconstruction with vascularized tissue (**Fig. 8**). Particularly in the head and neck and extremities, immediate reconstruction is required often to protect vital structures. Depending on the different treatment modalities, such as radiation and chemotherapy, reconstruction and wound healing can be affected adversely by these adjuncts in cancer therapy.

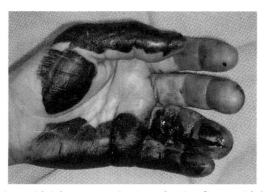

Fig. 6. Paint gun injury with ink extravasation into the ring finger with laceration.

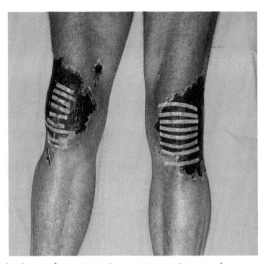

Fig. 7. Frostbite of the knees from excessive postoperative cryotherapy.

Wound Infection

Wound infection generally occurs when the bacterial count in the wound exceeds 10^5 bacteria per gram of tissue. This correlation of a critical number of bacteria was based on a study of quantitative burn wound biopsies that predicted skin graft failure.[6] Whether the infection remains localized to the wound, spreads to adjacent tissues, or becomes systemic is dependent on the interaction between the invading microbes and the host defenses.

Bacteria may gain entrance into skin and soft tissue directly, through dry or macerated skin to initiate a problem wound, or may convert an existing simple, acute wound into a chronic, complex wound (**Fig. 9**). Infection impairs the ability of the wound to heal by several mechanisms. All phases of the wound-healing cascade are affected by infection.[7] Infection decreases tissue Po_2 and prolongs the inflammatory phase. Significant infection (>10^5 bacteria) impairs leukocyte chemotaxis and migration, phagocytosis, and intracellular killing. Bacterial colonization impairs angiogenesis and epithelialization.[8,9] Lastly, microbial-derived collagenase breaks down the collagen in the wound, resulting in decreased wound strength and contraction. Factors to consider when managing an infected wound are the source of the bacteria,

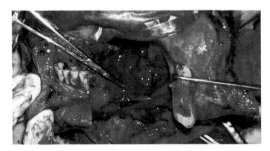

Fig. 8. View of a hemiglossectomy and floor-of-mouth defect requiring immediate reconstruction with free-tissue transfer.

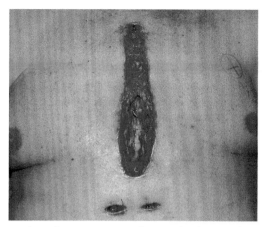

Fig. 9. Typical presentation of an acute sternal wound infection that only will heal with sound principles of debridement and vascularized soft tissue coverage.

rate of microbial proliferation, pathogenicity (endo/exotoxin production), and bacterial resistance.

MANAGEMENT
Timing

The "golden period" for the treatment of the acute wound has been defined at 6 hours. This is based on laboratory and clinical studies on the doubling time of bacterial colonization progressing to an invasive infection and from clinical outcomes describing the decreased risk for infection after debridement within that window of time.[10,11] An acute, open wound requires an initial "washout" to debride necrotic tissue and to reduce bacterial inoculation. Depending on the degree of contamination, tissue necrosis, and involved anatomy, the timing of the initial debridement is vital, because this can be the difference between future success or failure in wound closure.

This "golden period" before initial debridement needs to be separated from the concept of acute wound closure. In the late 1980s, Godina[12] expounded the concept of "emergency free flaps" for lower extremity reconstruction within the first 72 hours. This concept has its advantages with early wound closure and high success rates; however, there is a growing body of literature that supports staged debridement and reconstruction with equally high success rates.

The golden period serves as a guideline to acute wound treatment, but practical realities (eg, operating room time, delayed presentation) may impede this principle. These situations have opened the door to new techniques to optimize this time period[13] and to challenge the 6-hour dogma. The advent of antimicrobial silver dressings (eg, Acticoat) and negative pressure therapy (eg, vacuum assisted closure) will lead the way to the new and better use of technology to improve acute wound management.

Assessment/Exploration

The simple, acute wound, such as a laceration of skin and subcutaneous tissue, can be irrigated and closed primarily. Depending on the potential injury to other anatomic structures and the degree of contamination requiring special instrumentation, these simple lacerations can be treated in the office or emergency room.

When the acute wound involves underlying structures, is too large to close primarily, and requires special instrumentation, proper exploration with a full delineation of the anatomy and extent of injury is required in the operating room setting. The exploration includes defining the extent of the injury (zone of injury), the identification of key anatomic structures, and defining the extent of infection or necrosis.

At the skin and subcutaneous level, the edges need to be examined for vascularity and the amount of undermining determined. Nonviable skin appears dusky without capillary refill and does not bleed with excision. Subcutaneous fat should appear yellow and globular. Necrotic fat is dull in appearance and is gray/brown to black in color. Adjuncts to assessment include fluorescein dye, dermofluorometry, surface temperature readings, photoplethysmography, ultrasound Doppler flowmeters, laser Doppler, and transcutaneous Po_2 monitors. Fluorescein has proven to be a consistent and reliable method to determine skin viability.[14] Obtaining clear exposure of the underlying anatomy by enlarging the wound should be of high priority. Designing incisions to preserve blood supply to the skin and creating flaps over vital structures with reconstruction in mind will lead to simpler flap options for closure.

Muscles should be explored and tested for viability. Compartment syndrome should be considered, and aggressive fasciotomy should be the rule rather than the afterthought. Fascia is shiny white and surrounds skeletal muscle. If skeletal muscle bulges significantly after incising the fascia, it likely needs full decompression. Skeletal muscle is dull red, contractile, and vascular. Lack of contraction when stimulated, lack of bleeding, or a dark red color is a sign of necrosis. Tendons should be identified and tagged as necessary for future repair. Tendons are poorly vascularized and, thus, have the potential to become infected. Healthy tendons appear shiny white and are covered by paratenon. Tendon without paratenon easily can become necrotic.

Blood vessels should be tagged, not coagulated, for potential repair or used as future recipient vessels. Vessels greater than 1.5 mm in diameter may serve as a bridge to future reconstruction. Nerves also should be identified and tagged for primary repair or for future grafting.

Bone should be assessed and checked for viability. Bone is hard and white if healthy. Cortical bone is covered with periosteum, which is richly vascularized. Bone with periosteum will form granulation tissue and accept skin grafts, whereas bone without periosteum will not promote healing. Bone devoid of periosteum becomes an entrance point for infection and requires debridement and coverage with vascularized tissue.

In the extremity, a tourniquet should be used judiciously to have proximal control of blood vessels and turned up only after the full vascular examination of tissues has been complete.

Wound Culture

Swab culture of the open wound is a simple technique to obtain information about bacterial colonization and subsequent speciation and sensitivity testing to tailor appropriate antibiotic coverage. Swab cultures cannot determine the level of infection in a given tissue and has been criticized for not being adequate in this regard; however, it is still the most common method used and has high clinical usefulness.

Quantitative cultures also can be taken of the wound. This became used in the late 1960s with the seminal work of Robson and colleagues,[15] who determined improved sensitivity and specificity in predicting secondary wound closure. This work laid the groundwork for the understanding of bacterial bioburden in all soft tissues, including bone,[16] and more accurate determination of wound bed viability before closure.

Quantitative cultures have advantages, particularly in burn and indeterminate soft tissue infections, but they may have practical limitations based on individual institutions.

History of Wound Debridement

The history of wound debridement follows the course of surgical history. Understanding the history of wound treatments allows one to appreciate the advances in reconstructive plastic surgery. This is an exciting time for surgical treatment of wounds from a basic science and surgical standpoint. Further developments in the history are covered elsewhere in this issue.

Principles of Debridement

Debridement is the most fundamental principle in surgical wound bed preparation before closure. Inadequate debridement is the surgical corollary to a postoperative infectious complication after acute wound bed closure. – Plastic surgery dictum

Operative wound debridement must be systematic and thorough, working simultaneously with the wound exploration. Preoperative radiographs should be considered if bony involvement or if complex deeper anatomy is suspected. Abscess cavities should be drained adequately. Tissue viability needs to be determined with examination of the color, temperature, and presence of bleeding. Debridement involves the removal of devitalized, infected, or necrotic tissue from the wound. At the completion of the debridement, "no stone should be left unturned," and every crevice and adjacent anatomy of the wound should be known.

At the heart of the debridement is the surgeon's knowledge of the anatomy and one's skill with instrumentation to remove nonviable tissue. Debridement to bleeding tissues serves as the end point for most tissues, but specialized tissue, such as cartilage, tendon, and irradiated wounds, often requires experienced judgment and careful consideration. Multiple operative wound debridements may be necessary to achieve wound stability depending on the necrotic and infectious bioburden.

Debridement and immediate closure of the acute wound is the main goal for selected wounds without intrinsic, mechanical, or extrinsic deficiency.[1] A definitive one-step procedure limits the patient to one anesthesia, reduces desiccation of the wound, shortens hospital stay, reduces cost, and is extremely valuable if vital structures are exposed within the wound. Sequential debridement is important when there is an inability to accurately predict the amount of nonviable tissue and extent of debridement required at the initial operation. This allows one to define the exact margins of the wound, potentially preserving borderline tissue surrounding the wound as well as allowing cultures to be collected and processed before wound closure. In this situation, sequential wound debridement and wound observation are important. Over the course of serial debridements, wound biopsies with quantitative cultures may be obtained to assess the status of bacterial invasion.

INSTRUMENTS FOR DEBRIDEMENT
Sharp Debridement

Sharp debridement remains the standard of surgical debridement. It is classically performed with the scalpel blade or scissors removing tissue in sections, usually outside the interface between the wound margin and normal tissue (ie, excising a margin of normal tissue). The scalpel can come in multiple shapes and sizes, such as a Weck knife, which can tangentially excise tissue. Curettes are an adjunct to sharp debridement using a scraping action on the tissue. Often, granulation tissue, bone, and smaller crevices are amenable to the curette. Rongeurs and osteotomes are designed to excise tougher tissue in large bites or with osteotomies. In combination, the surgeon has a vast array of tools from which to choose to obtain a viable wound bed (**Fig. 10**).

Irrigating Systems

Irrigating systems are used often in acute wounds with a large bacterial load, before and after surgery. They provide a way to nonsurgically debride and cleanse the wound with saline or antibiotic irrigation. Irrigation to remove debris and lessen bacterial contamination (dilution) is an essential component of open fracture care.[17] Intraoperative irrigation is applied with high pressure (2–10 psi), whereas it is used postoperatively to cleanse chronic wounds gently to control the antimicrobial load. The volume of the irrigation fluid is an important factor because increased volume improves the wound cleansing and decreases the bacterial load. High-pressure flow also was shown to remove more bacteria and debris, thus lowering the rate of wound infection, compared with low-pressure irrigation.[18] Pulsatile flow is used often for debridement of necrotic tissue and was shown experimentally to remove bacteria more efficiently than continuous pressure flow (**Fig. 11**). Irrigation in its multiple forms serves as an adjunct to sharp surgical debridement. Controversy surrounds its effectiveness when its parameters for volume, pressure, and antimicrobial additions are discussed. Other concerns, such as further bacterial spread and contamination, underscore the importance of adequate sharp debridement before pulse irrigation.

Debridement by Hydrocision

Hydrocision (Versajet, Smith and Nephew, Largo, Florida) has entered the foray of tools in surgical debridement.[19] By simultaneously cutting and removing tissue with water through a high-pressure opening, it acts as an ideal debridement tool. In our experience, the Versajet has clear advantages over the current methods of soft tissue debridement in its precision, efficiency, and clinical usefulness. It is particularly useful in concavities (eg, pressure ulcers and joint spaces) and in tight spaces (eg, breast capsules). Its impact has been significant in burns. Its usefulness on bone has yet to be determined, but there is promising data from the European experience on its use with orthopedic hardware and intramedullary bony debridement.[20]

Dressings

Between the stages of wound management, multiple dressings are available to address its various characteristics, most importantly bacteria and fluid exudate. In

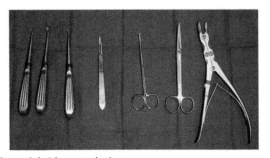

Fig. 10. Standard sharp debridement devices.

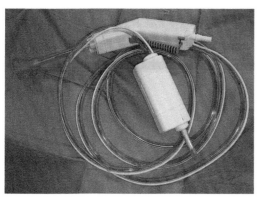

Fig. 11. Pulse lavage.

this regard, several dressings, which include negative pressure therapy and antimicrobial dressings, have made a major impact in the past decade.

Both of these therapies are covered in more detail in separate articles elsewhere in this issue; suffice it to say that the advances in wound management with these two concepts have created healing environments that provide improved comfort and efficacy for patient and care provider, by decreasing pain and the number of dressing changes.

Negative pressure therapy and antimicrobial dressings play a major role as a bridge to reconstruction. If used appropriately and in a timely fashion, these adjuncts can impact acute wound management significantly; however, we have begun to see basic principles of wound management ignored, and more practitioners are using these therapeutics as a panacea to wounds, with disastrous consequences (**Figs. 12–14**).

RECONSTRUCTION OF THE ACUTE WOUND
Plastic Surgery and the Reconstructive Ladder

The reconstructive ladder (**Fig. 15**) is a useful way to plan the closure of any wound systematically. It is a logical sequence to regain form and function as the anatomy of the defect dictates. It is important to remember that the ladder is a guideline to

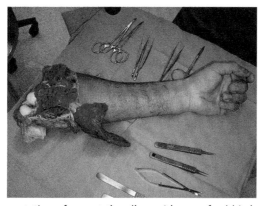

Fig. 12. Complete amputation of arm at the elbow. 4 hours of cold ischemia.

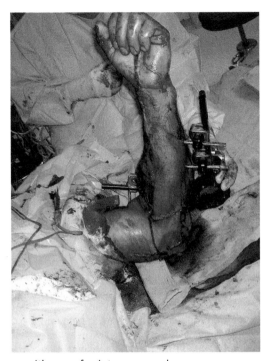

Fig. 13. Replanted arm with open fasciotomy wounds.

reconstruction, and, in some instances, moving up and down the ladder also can result in wound closure. Each case should be looked at on an individual basis, understanding the host factors and the anatomy of the wound to dictate the best option for closure.

Reconstructive options begin simply and become more complex as needed for a given defect. The first and most straightforward approach is to allow the wound to close spontaneously after an adequate debridement, allowing the wound to form granulation tissue and "heal from the inside out." A common example of this technique is after an open laparotomy, which would be considered a clean, contaminated wound after bowel spillage, closing the fascia but packing the wound until closure. The advantages of this method lie in its simplicity and avoidance of a closed wound infection. Disadvantages include an extended time period to healing, dressing changes, and a suboptimal scar.

Moving up the ladder, the second method of treatment is by primary closure of the wound. This is used most commonly in a simple laceration, which can be repaired in its anatomic layers. Primary closure is the preferred method of closure for any acute wound. Primary repair of injured structures, such as the skin, nerve, tendon, and blood vessels, is the preferred approach when the zone of injury is small and the wound is clean (**Fig. 16**). Tension, potential infection, and indeterminate zone of injury preclude primary closure. The advantages of this method are its simplicity and best healing potential with correct anatomic alignment. The disadvantages include potential wound infection and the need for advanced surgical technique to repair the involved structures.

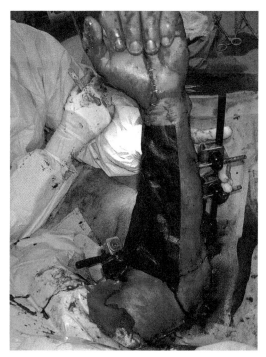

Fig. 14. Open fasciotomy wounds covered with Acticoat antimicrobial dressing, which allowed comfort for the patient (dressing change on the third day) and less work for the nursing staff, obviating dressing changes two to three times per day.

Plastic Surgery and the Reconstructive Ladder

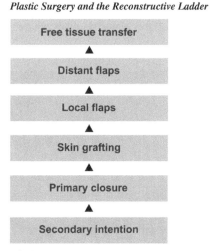

Fig. 15. The reconstructive ladder—a stepwise, systematic approach to the closure of the acute wound.

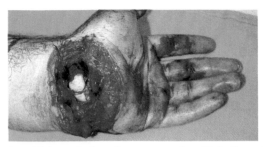

Fig. 16. Spaghetti wrist with lacerated median nerve and multiple flexor tendons in need of primary repair.

If the defect cannot be closed primarily, then the next step is the placement of a skin graft (**Fig. 17**). Because a graft requires its underlying bed to supply the nutrients and ultimate blood supply, the wound bed must be clean and viable. This requires meticulous wound bed preparation, hemostasis, and appropriate dressings to protect the graft. The advantages of this method include its technical simplicity and quick closure of the wound without the creation of flaps. The disadvantages lie in its need for meticulous wound bed preparation, potential poor esthetics, contour defects, and poor durability as compared with a local flap.

Local tissue rearrangement and local flaps are the next step up the ladder. Local tissue rearrangement may involve creation of small geometric flap designs that can be random pattern flaps or larger flap designs based on axial circulation. Local flaps can take any layer of the soft tissue and can be combined to rotate or transpose for wound closure (**Fig. 18**). Examples of local flaps include fasciocutaneous flaps, musculocutaneous flaps, fascial flaps with skin graft, and composite flaps with bone and skin. The advantages of the local flaps include their blood supply, similarity to the surrounding tissue, and tissue durability. Disadvantages include the need for a more complex operation and a small zone of injury, which does not include the flap to be elevated.

The value of vascularized muscle in more complex wounds has been defined well. Muscle flaps or musculocutaneous flaps should be considered the gold standard, because they are bulky, able to fill large defects, obliterate dead space, are malleable,

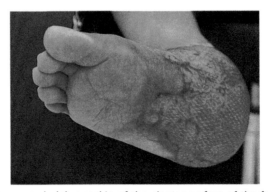

Fig. 17. Contrast the normal glabrous skin of the plantar surface of the foot with a meshed skin graft on a muscle flap for subtotal foot resurfacing after a degloving injury.

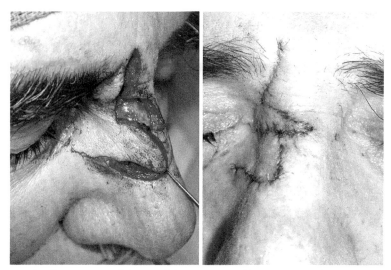

Fig. 18. Basal cell carcinoma of the nasal dorsum excised leaving a significant defect. Bilobe flap designed allowing complete closure of defect.

and are well vascularized. The well-vascularized muscle flap provides stable coverage and serves as a delivery system for leukocytes, oxygen, and antibiotics.[21]

Local tissue expansion is a modification of the local tissue option (**Fig. 19**). Skin and soft tissue adjacent to the defect are the preferred tissues for closure because of the similarity in skin color, texture, and contour. The size, location, or the zone of injury may preclude the use of adjacent tissue for expansion, particularly in the acute setting; however, tissue expansion does have a role in a secondary procedure. For example, a wound may be treated with a skin graft initially and allowed to heal. The surrounding skin is then expanded at a secondary procedure, and, ultimately, the skin graft is excised and the expanded tissue is used to cover the defect.

Free-tissue transfer is the most complex method whereby the acute wound can be closed. This technique has all of the advantages of the local flap with the added benefit of transferring the tissue anywhere on the body by way of microsurgical anastomoses.

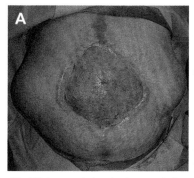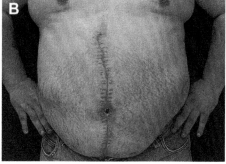

Fig. 19. (*A*) Large abdominal wound closed with skin graft; 300-cm^3 tissue expanders are in place bilaterally in preparation to excise skin graft and close primarily. (*B*) Two months postoperatively from tissue expander removal and closure of abdominal wound.

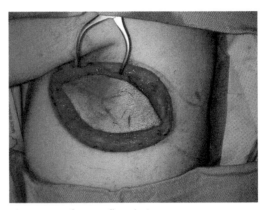

Fig. 20. Thoracodorsal artery perforator flap design.

Free flaps can be designed to include multiple tissue types (eg, skin, muscle, tendon, fascia, bone, nerve) and can be dissected to include only the tissues required for reconstruction (perforator flaps), which can reduce donor site morbidity (**Figs. 20 and 21**). They can be prelaminated and prefabricated for added complexity in reconstruction.[22,23] Free-tissue transfer allows for a one-step operation of the most complex wounds. Oncologic defects frequently require free-tissue transfer because the local tissues are not suitable for reconstruction. Free flap success rates are well over 95% at microsurgical centers. It is not uncommon now to view free-tissue transfer as a first stop option in complex reconstruction, modifying the reconstructive ladder as the "reconstructive elevator"(**Fig. 22**).[24] The advantages of free-tissue transfer include its freedom in reconstruction for complex and specialized areas where local flaps are not available. Disadvantages include a more complex operation and the potential for vascular compromise.

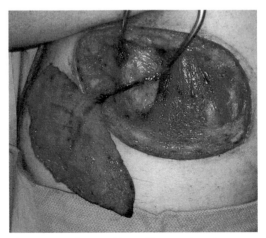

Fig. 21. Thoracodorsal artery perforator flap with a septocutaneous perforator (blue) in continuity with the thoracodorsal artery of the latissimus muscle. This flap is elevated with minimal donor site morbidity.

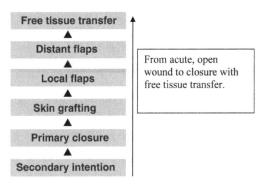

Fig. 22. The reconstructive elevator: an approach that bypasses the intermediate steps to ultimate closure.

SUMMARY

The acute wound presents a spectrum of issues that need to be considered before its ultimate closure. In the past decade, significant advances have been made in the area of debridement, dressings, and surgical options that allow the modern plastic surgeon to treat any wound of any complexity. We have entered the era of refinement in reconstructive plastic surgery such that form, function, and esthetic considerations are the ultimate goals in closing a wound. Throughout this, however, the principles of surgical wound management have remained steadfast.

REFERENCES

1. Hansen SL, Mathes SJ. Problem wounds and principles of closure. In: Plastic surgery. New York: Elsevier; 2006. p. 901–50.
2. Alexander JW, Gottschlich MM. Nutritional immunomodulation in burn patients. Crit Care Med 1990;18:S149–53.
3. Goldstein EJC. Management of human and animal bite wounds. J Am Acad Dermatol 1989;21:1275–9.
4. Smith PF, Meadowcroft AM, May DB. Treating mammalian bite wounds. J Clin Pharm Ther 2000;25:85–9.
5. Lee CK, Pardun J, Buntic R, et al. Severe frostbite of the knees after cryotherapy. Orthopedics 2007;30(1):63–4.
6. Robson MC. Infection in the surgical patient: an imbalance in the normal equilibrium. Clin Plast Surg 1979;6:493–501.
7. Robson MC. Wound infection. A failure of wound healing caused by an imbalance of bacteria. Surg Clin North Am 1997;77:637–45.
8. Hunt TK. Disorders of wound healing. World J Surg 1980;4:271–85.
9. Gottrup F, Firmin R, Hunt TK, et al. The dynamic properties of tissue oxygen in healing flaps. Surgery 1984;95:527–36.
10. Hoover NW, Ivins JC. Wound debridement. Arch Surg 1959;79:701–10.
11. Kinsfater K, Jonassen EA. Osteomyelitis in grade II and III open tibial fractures with late debridement. J Orthop Trauma 1995;9(2):121–7.
12. Godina M. A thesis on the management of injuries to the lower extremity. Ljubljana (Slovenia): Presernova Druzba Publishing House; 1991.
13. Suk M. Debridement of acute traumatic wounds. In: Surgical wound healing and management. New York: Informa Healthcare USA, Inc; 2007. p. 69–82.

14. Sloan GM, Reinisch JF. Flap physiology and the prediction of flap viability. Hand Clin 1985;1:609–19.
15. Robson M, Heggers JP. Bacterial quantification of open wounds. Mil Med 1969; 134(1):19–24.
16. Heller WA, Gottlieb LJ, Zachary LS, et al. The use of quantitative bacteriologic assessment of bone. Plast Reconstr Surg 1997;100(2):397–401.
17. Dirschl DR, Duff GP, Dahners LE, et al. High pressure pulsatile irrigation of intra-articular fractures: effects on fracture healing. J Orthop Trauma 1998;12:460–6.
18. Burgess AR, Poka A, Brumback RJ, et al. Pedestrian tibial injuries. J Trauma 1987;27:596–604.
19. Klein M, Hunter S, Heimbach D, et al. The Versajet water dissector: a new tool for tangential excision. J Burn Care Rehabil 2007;26(6):483–7.
20. Davidson JS, Toh EM. Debridement of infected orthopedic prostheses. In: Surgical wound healing and management. New York: Informa Healthcare USA; 2007. p. 131–40.
21. Calderon W, Chang N, Mathes SJ. Comparison of the effect of bacterial inoculation in musculocutaneous and fasciocutaneous flaps. Plast Reconstr Surg 1986; 77(5):785–94.
22. Pribaz JJ, Fine NA. Prefabricated and prelaminated flaps for head and neck reconstruction. Clin Plast Surg 2001;28(2):261–72, vii.
23. Walton RL, Burget GC, Beahm EK. Microsurgical reconstruction of the nasal lining [case reports]. Plast Reconstr Surg 2005;115(7):1813–29.
24. Gottlieb LJ, Krieger LM. From the reconstructive ladder to the reconstructive elevator. Plast Reconstr Surg 1994;93(7):1503–4.

Benign Skin Lesions: Lipomas, Epidermal Inclusion Cysts, Muscle and Nerve Biopsies

Kartik A. Pandya, MD[a],*, Frederick Radke, MD, FACS[b,c]

KEYWORDS

- Lipomas • Epidermal inclusion cysts • Muscle
- Nerve biopsies

LIPOMAS AND EPIDERMAL INCLUSION CYSTS
Overview

Common surgical procedures done in the minor operating room or in the office include removal of lumps, bumps, and biopsies. Removal of superficial masses and epidermal cysts is frequently performed at the request of patients for cosmetic purposes, but is occasionally done due to diagnostic insecurity. These lesions include benign and malignant varieties as well as solid and cystic lesions.

Lipomas are benign skin tumors composed of mature fat cells and are the most common subcutaneous tumors.[1] Although many of these can be removed in the surgical clinic or minor operating room, some require more advanced preoperative planning and more complicated resection. The diagnosis, pathology, and treatment of benign tumors, and other commonly associated tumors that may require a more substantial workup and operative intervention, are discussed.

Epidermal inclusion cysts are benign skin lesions that arise from obstructed or ruptured pilosebaceous follicles that can also be excised locally.[2] In some cases an associated infection or foreign body reaction can occur if the cyst contents are spilled into the surrounding tissues, and therefore their treatment is slightly different from that of simple lipomas.[3] Epidermal inclusion cysts are also known as sebaceous, epithelial, keratin, and epidermoid cysts.[2] The term sebaceous cyst is commonly used but is inaccurate due to the absence of sebum within the cyst. The term used here is *epidermal inclusion cyst*.

[a] Department of Surgery, Maine Medical Center, Maine Surgical Care Group, 22 Bramhall Street, Portland, ME 04102, USA
[b] University of Vermont College of Medicine, Burlington, VT 05405, USA
[c] Surgical Services, Mercy Hospital, 144 State Street, Portland, ME 04102, USA
* Corresponding author.
E-mail address: pandyk@mmc.org (K.A. Pandya).

Surg Clin N Am 89 (2009) 677–687
doi:10.1016/j.suc.2009.03.002
0039-6109/09/$ – see front matter © 2009 Elsevier Inc. All rights reserved.
surgical.theclinics.com

Other minor procedures such as nerve and muscle biopsies may be performed to diagnose neuromuscular diseases.

Diagnosis

Lipomatous masses include simple lipomas, angiolipomas, well-differentiated lipomas, and liposarcomas. Another variant, the "atypical lipoma," is also noted in the literature, with histologic similarities to the well-differentiated liposarcoma and propensity for local recurrence.

Complicated lipomas include masses found on imaging to have multiple septae or involvement of deeper structures and nerve involvement. These are normally found to be well-differentiated lipomas, deep atypical lipomas, or liposarcomas.

Lipomas typically occur in the 40- to 60-year-old age group, but they can also occur in young children. Lipomas usually present as slow-growing masses without symptoms of pain or functional impairment. The incidence of lipomas is cited to be 2.1 per 1000 individuals.[4] Lipomas are multiple approximately 5% of the time.[5]

Patients presenting with a subcutaneous lipoma typically do not receive preoperative imaging. In cases of large lipomas (>5 cm), those irregular in shape, and those with symptoms of myofascial involvement, imaging is warranted using ultrasound, computed tomography (CT), or magnetic resonance imaging (MRI). Imaging should also be obtained if the tissue biopsy indicates the presence of an infiltrating mass.

MRI is the most sensitive imaging modality for lipomatous masses and has a high negative predictive value. On MRI, the fatty nature of the lipoma elicits a strong T1 signal; however, a large lipoma could be difficult to differentiate from a well-differentiated liposarcoma.[6] MRI can be useful in the diagnosis of benign lipomas. Studies show a high positive predictive value for benign simple lipomas. The main criteria for determining a simple lipoma from more complicated masses are the presence of enhancing septae, nonadipose areas, and high T2 signal within the lesion. Gaskin and Helms[7] report the difficulties associated with predicting well-differentiated liposarcoma from benign lesions, with the tendency to "over call" the lesion as a more aggressive entity.

Indications for removal of a lipoma typically include cosmetic concerns, but these tumors can also cause nerve impingement, pain, and consequent functional limitations that necessitate removal (such as with angiolipomas). Other indications for removal of lipomas include increase in size, irregular characteristics (induration), size (>5 cm), samples of core needle biopsy consistent with atypical features, or other features more consistent with a sarcoma (invasion/involvement of deep fascia).[8]

Differential diagnosis of lipomas includes epidermal inclusion cyst, hematoma, vasculitis, panniculitis, rheumatic nodules, metastatic cancer/subcutaneous tumor, or infections.[9]

Epidermal inclusion cysts also present as benign slow-growing masses but can also rupture before the patient seeks treatment. If the keratin-filled cyst ruptures, an intense foreign body giant cell reaction can occur, leading to pain and further swelling.[5] Epidermal inclusion cysts have been associated with Gardner syndrome and individuals with extensive cysts should prompt a gastrointestinal neoplasm workup.

Classification

A simple lipoma may be watched clinically or removed in accordance with patient preference. The more invasive and histologic atypical lesions such as "atypical" lipoma, well-differentiated lipomas, and liposarcomas should be removed due to mass effects and, in the case of the liposarcoma, due to the propensity for systemic disease.[8]

There are multiple classification schemes for lipomas depending on the anatomic location (face/back versus trunk/extremities). Lipomas can be classified in different morphologic categories, such as lipoma, angiolipoma, well-differentiated lipoma, and liposarcoma. Closely related tumors composed of immature fat cells and mature brown fat cells include lipoblastomas and hibernomas, respectively.[10] Others classify lipomas as simple lipomas, fibrolipomas, angiolipomas, spindle cell lipomas, myelolipomas, and pleomorphic lipomas.[11] Lipoblastomas are either circumscribed or diffuse and composed of immature adipocytes. They typically occur in the infant population and can histologically resemble a form of liposarcomas.[12] Hibernomas are circumscribed tumors composed of mature brown fat tumors and histologically resemble fatty tumors in hibernating animals.[12] Lipomas can also be broken down into simple lipomas and pleomorphic lipomas. Pleomorphic lipomas are more common on the neck and might require tissue sampling to arrive at the proper diagnosis.[13] It is important to distinguish whether the lipoma is singular or one of multiple lesions, and to discern the presence of an associated syndrome. The subsequent histopathology will determine further follow-up with a more advanced surgical excision or referral to surgical oncology.

Syndromes associated with lipomas include adiposis dolorosa, benign symmetric lipomatosis (Madelung syndrome), Bannayan-Riley-Ruvalcaba syndrome, and Gardner syndrome, among others.[9,14,15]

Adiposis dolorosa is a genetic condition whereby patients present with multiple painful lipomas, and has a higher prevalence in women. This is sometimes misdiagnosed as simply a sporadic occurrence of multiple lipomas or neurofibromatosis.[16]

Benign symmetric lipomatosis, also known as Madelung disease, is a rare disorder affecting mostly men of Mediterranean descent. Patients develop significantly enlarged lipomatous masses that can be debilitating. Treatment consists of staged surgical resection and liposuction.[17]

Cowden syndrome includes hamartomas affecting all three germ lines. These tumors can affect the endocrine (thyroid), skin (breast), and reproductive systems (endometrium).[18]

Gardner syndrome is described as thyroid nodules, multiple epidermal inclusion cysts, osteomas, and intestinal polyposis. Recently it has been shown that the presence of intestinal polyps is required for an accurate diagnosis.[19]

In cases of childhood lipomas, attention must be paid to the rest of the physical examination due to the higher incidence of associated developmental abnormalities. The syndromal states associated with lipomas in children include Bannayan-Riley-Ruvalcaba syndrome (BRRS) or Cowden syndrome, which are both associated with PTEN gene mutations.[18,20] A child with associated classic BRRS findings of macrocephaly, hemangiomas, and speckled penis should warrant a more thorough genetic workup.

The epidermal inclusion cyst classification also includes other related entities such as trichilemmal cysts, milia, and steatocystoma multiplex. Although all result from obstruction of the pilosebaceous follicle, there are important histologic differences.[5]

Histopathology

Fatty tumors are classified histologically according to their composition. The most immature fatty cell tumors are known as lipoblastomas, whereas tumors composed of brown fat are called hibernomas. A mature white fat tumor is known as a lipoma.[10] Simple lipomas have a thick, well-defined capsule that is distinctly separate from the surrounding tissue. The location of lipomas can be varied, as they can be subcutaneous or invade the myofascial layers and be intimately associated with muscle and soft tissue. Further histologic subclassification of the lipoma depends on the tissue depth and involvement of other structures.

Spindle cell lipomas and pleomorphic lipomas are associated with dorsal, head, and neck distribution and histologically have collagen-forming spindle cells interspersed with adipocytes. Angiolipomas are composed of adipocytes with a vascular infiltration and are more commonly associated with pain and multiplicity, compared with other types of lipomas.[12]

Lipomas of the extremities are classified according to their involvement of subcutaneous and deep dermal tissues. For example, a lipoma involving the tendon sheath is classified as a synovium-related lipoma with tendon sheath involvement.[10]

Epidermal inclusion cysts consist of stratified epithelium-lined cysts filled with keratin. Trichilemmal cysts are also composed of keratin but lack the granular layer found in epidermal inclusion cysts and are more often found on the scalp. Milia are essentially miniature epidermal inclusion cysts that are also found in eccrine sweat glands. Steatocystoma multiplex are cysts filled with sebum and sebaceous glands.[5]

Genetics

Lipomas occur in an isolated fashion or as a part of syndromes. The most commonly seen lipomas are typically isolated lesions not associated with any generalized malady. The genetics for lipomas are variable with respect to associated syndromes. With BRRS, there is an association with the MEN1 (Multiple Endocrine Neoplasia 1) and PTEN (Phosphatase and Tensin homolog, deleted on chromosome 10) genes.[21,22] These genes are part of the hamartoma tumor syndromes. Other genetic associations with lipomas include 12q14-15, 6p, 13q (for simple lipomas), and 16q and 13q (for spindle cell and pleomorphic lipomas).[11] It is commonly accepted that a sarcomatous differentiation occurs in about 1% of simple lipomas.[23]

Epidermal inclusion cysts have been associated with Gardner syndrome but related entities such as pilar cysts or steatocystoma multiplex are not.[24] Leppard[25] found that approximately 53% of patients with Gardner syndrome have epidermal inclusion cysts.

Medical Treatment

Historically, treatment of lipomas has consisted of surgical excision, but advances in medical treatment have allowed for reduction in lipoma size. Most treatments have centered on steroid injections to shrink the lipomas. A small case series has shown an approximately 75% reduction in lesion size with 2 to 3 injections of deoxycholate. This is different from prior experience with the commercially available phosphatidylcholine and deoxycholate mixtures used to inject and shrink lipomas.[15]

Epidermal inclusion cysts will not regress with nonsurgical treatment. However, in cases of infected cysts, some have described infiltration with corticosteroids and delayed surgical excision. This method is not commonly employed.[3,25]

Surgical Treatment

Surgical treatment of lipomas involves simple excision. In many uncomplicated cases (those without soft tissue infiltration or excessive size), the excision can be performed in the office or the minor procedures room under local anesthetic. The surgical approach involves maintaining the normal aesthetic contours of the skin, however different approaches and incisions are used on the face versus trunk/thigh, and there is debate on whether an elliptical or a punch biopsy incision is more appropriate. It is our recommendation to use an elliptical incision for the most complete excision and best cosmetic outcome.[26]

After anesthetizing the skin with a local anesthetic, an overlying skin incision is made approximately one half to three quarters the length of the lipoma along Langer lines (defined as parallel skin creases correlating with the direction of least elasticity). It helps to mark the border of the lipoma before dissection. Using a blunt and sharp dissection technique, the fibrous capsule is separated from the surrounding soft tissue. Care must be taken not to invade the capsule to maintain proper aesthetics. Bleeding is controlled with electrocautery. The wound is approximated with absorbable subcutaneous sutures and overlying subcuticular sutures or skin adhesive. The most common postoperative complications include hematomas and seromas, which can be locally managed and usually require aspiration at most.[4]

Alternative techniques, including minimal-scar segmental extraction of lipomas, have been described for larger/multiple lipomas.[4] This technique uses segmental dissection of the lipoma to facilitate removal from a small incision.

Another technique involves liposuction of lipomas if they are found to be histologically benign; however, this technique is not associated with the best aesthetic outcome.[27,28]

For more advanced tumors involving the deep fascia or muscle, advanced operative planning is required, including imaging with MRI or CT scans.

Several different surgical procedures are used for excision of epidermal inclusion cysts. A small incision is often made over the lesion and the cyst cavity entered to allow expression of the keratin contents. After thorough expression by digital pressure the cyst wall is excised. In contrast to lipomas, a retained cyst wall will more often result in cyst recurrence. As mentioned earlier, there is also a propensity for a significant foreign body reaction if cyst contents are expressed into the surrounding tissues. Bacterial infections can also complicate cyst excision as they make the cyst wall more friable. Common organisms include aerobic and anaerobic flora, specifically *Staphylococcus,* group A *Streptococcus*, *Escherichia coli*, and anaerobes such as *Peptostreptococcus* and *Bacteroides*. The cyst wall itself varies in thickness and therefore ease of manipulation and removal depend on the cyst location; facial cysts have thinner walls compared with scalp/body cysts.[2,5] Others have described excision via punch biopsies of cysts as large as 1 to 2 cm.[26] For more complicated or larger cysts, a wider excision to ensure cyst wall removal is required and therefore is associated with a greater cosmetic defect.

It has been traditionally taught that infected epidermal inclusion cysts should be incised and drained much like an abscess and then later resected, and any surgical intervention should be delayed until after the inflammation subsides. However, more recent studies show that, with primary resection, lavage, and proper wound care, infected cysts can be safely excised with a lower recurrence rate. It awaits further scientific validation before a widespread recommendation to close an incision in an infected field can be adopted.[29]

The long axis should be along skin lines and the short axis perpendicular to create an elliptical incision. A length to width ratio of 3:1 is used to construct the ellipse. Next, local anesthetic with or without epinephrine is used to form a wheal and anesthetize the skin. A blade is used to enter the dermis but avoid the cyst wall. Using tenotomy scissors, retraction, and blunt dissection, the cyst is removed along with the overlying skin. Care must be taken to ensure hemostasis and that wound closure can proceed with a single layered closure in the cases of small 1- to 2-cm cysts; larger defects will require placement of deep dermal absorbable sutures.[30] Infected cysts that are symptomatic can be incised and drained with a small overlying incision and gentle manual evacuation of the cyst contents.

Surgical sites on the face are aesthetically the most important. In planning excision of lesions on the face (lipomas or epidermal inclusion cysts), additional evaluation of facial furrows along with skin lines should be performed. The facial furrow might preclude a separate larger incision, however the surgeon may be able to place his incision within the furrow in a "distant" fashion and still excise the lesion.[31]

Trichilemmal cysts (also known as scalp cysts or "wen's") are cysts that materialize from the outer root sheath of hair follicles. Their excision is similar to that of epidermal inclusion cysts; however, if a related entity known as a proliferating trichilemmal tumor (PTT) is present, the excision is slightly different. In cases of PTT, a 1-cm margin is used for excision, and these lesions are also appropriate for Mohs procedure.[32] Proliferating trichilemmal tumors are larger than trichilemmal cyst counterparts; however, the definitive diagnosis is made during histopathology. Because the correct diagnosis might not be known at the time of the procedure, re-excision might be required to obtain 1-cm margins.

Because malignant skin lesions can be diagnosed grossly as benign, excised lesions should be sent to histopathology. Although this step has fallen out of favor, even experienced surgeons and dermatologists may occasionally classify a malignant lesion as benign. It is therefore advisable to send all biopsied tissues to pathology.[33]

Recurrence

The local recurrence rate of simple lipomas involving subcutaneous tissue is approximately 1% to 2%.[12] There is a general consensus that recurrence of simple lipomas is not affected by wide resection or simply "coring out" the lesion. The risk of local recurrence is greatest with intramuscular lipomas at 19%.[5] In the case of well-differentiated liposarcomas, the risk of local recurrence increases with marginal resection, with a reported rate of approximately 50% and a median time postresection of 5 years in patients with marginal resections. Wide resection of well-differentiated liposarcomas decreases the risk of recurrence but is associated with greater morbidity.

The recurrence rate of epidermal inclusion cysts is approximately 3% irrespective of punch biopsy or cyst invasion/expression/excision method, although others have reported a slightly lower rate of recurrence with a wide/elliptical excision.[26]

Discussion

Simple lipomas can be safely excised under local anesthetic in the surgeon's office or in the minor procedures room. Although most lipomas are not associated with a malignancy or syndromes states, these should be considered if dealing with children or if there are associated signs of a systemic disorder. Risk of local recurrence is low with most benign lipomas, however more aggressive and deeply rooted lipomas are associated with a significantly higher risk of recurrence. In cases of more advanced lipomas or those with troubling clinical and histologic features, operative planning and imaging are required.

Epidermal inclusion cysts require a more careful dissection to avoid an inflammatory reaction from spilled cyst contents and to decrease the recurrence rate from retained cyst wall. While the decision to perform a surgical excision versus a punch biopsy is dependent on surgeon preference, both techniques have been used successfully in their treatment.

MUSCLE AND NERVE BIOPSIES
Overview

Muscle and nerve biopsies are performed to diagnose inflammatory conditions resulting in myositis and neuropathy (peripheral or systemic). An overview of muscle and nerve biopsies is presented here, along with indications, contraindications, and technical aspects of the procedures.

Combined muscle and nerve biopsies are performed to diagnose isolated nerve vasculitis (nonsystemic vasculitic neuropathy) and systemic vasculitic neuropathy. Diagnosis has traditionally centered around biopsy of the vastus lateralis or peroneus brevis muscles and sural or superficial peroneal nerves. Recently, it has been shown there is no improved sensitivity in disease detection with combined muscle and nerve biopsies.[34]

Indications

Indications for muscle biopsies include differentiating primary muscular disorders (myopathy) from neurologic disorders (neuropathy), which often present as similar symptoms, and for the diagnosis of systemic immune disorders (**Table 1**).[35]

With advancements in genetic analysis, many of the more common "dystrophiopathies" no longer require muscle biopsy as an initial diagnostic mode. These conditions include Duchenne or Becker muscular dystrophy, myotonic dystrophy, periodic paralysis, and endocrine myopathy.

Tissue Selection and Technique

Biopsy samples from muscles should be obtained from symptomatic sites. For diffuse conditions, such as systemic vasculitis, the vastus lateralis is chosen. The basic technique of muscle biopsy is as follows.

After drawing an incision along a Langer line, the skin is infiltrated with a local anesthetic of the surgeon's choice; care should be taken not to inject below the dermis to prevent distortion of tissues. An incision is made along the line and the subcutaneous tissue dissected to the level of the fascia. The fascia is opened and a 1 cm by 0.5 cm by 0.5 cm section of muscle is removed. No monopolar cauterization should be used to prevent damaging the tissue and introducing artifacts in microscopic sections. The bleeding is stopped with digital pressure, packing, and suture ligature if required. The closure is performed in two layers to minimize dead space and prevent seroma accumulation. The skin is closed with absorbable suture in a subcuticular fashion in low-tension areas. The mattress suture is used in high-tension areas such as the shoulder (if a deltoid biopsy was performed).

Three samples should be obtained during the biopsy for fresh, fixed, and genetic/biochemical analysis. The amount of muscle removed can vary depending on whether the biopsy is being performed as an open procedure or a core needle biopsy. During the open procedure, samples approximately 1 cm long and 0.5 cm by 0.5 cm wide are obtained. In a core needle biopsy, the core size varies depending on the needle and is

Table 1	
Common indications/contraindications for muscle biopsies	
Indications	**Contraindications**
Muscular dystrophy (most)	Dystrophinopathies
Inflammatory myopathy	Myotonic
Steroid induced myopathy	Duchenne
Metabolic myopathy	Becker
	Limb girdle
	Periodic paralysis
	Endocrine myopathy

really only useful for biochemical markers and genetic analysis, without yielding significant morphologic tissue data.

Once the fresh sample is obtained, it is rushed to the laboratory using an ice-chilled bag on saline soaked gauze. A light microscopy slide is made from the fresh sample and the tissue stained with hematoxylin and eosin. Alternate stains to isolate proper protein production and function are outlined in **Table 2**.

The fixed (permanent) sample is used for electron microscopy and involves tissue that is approximately the same size as used in the fresh (frozen) section. The sample is stored in 4% paraformaldehyde and then subsequently immersed in gluteraldehyde.

Electron microscopy (EM) is a costly method to evaluate cellular structures at the molecular level. During the original muscle biopsy, a sample should be kept from the permanent section for EM. The process of fixation and preparation of EM samples is beyond the scope of this article but the initial steps are similar to fixation of the permanent sample.[35]

Findings and Follow-up

Muscle biopsies can also provide information to distinguish between primary neuropathies and myopathies. Primary neuropathies consist of nerve atrophy from numerous causes.

There are certain microscopic features that can help to distinguish a peripheral neuropathy from a myopathy including evidence of individual muscle fiber atrophy, regrouping of muscle fibers, renervation, and denervation.

The diagnosis of myopathies is only partly dependent on the tissue biopsy. At present there are numerous tests that can diagnose individual myopathies, including tests for Duchenne, Becker, and mitochondrial muscular dystrophies.

Findings of inflammation, helpful in the diagnosis of myositis, can also be present on the muscle biopsy.

Indications for Nerve Biopsy

Nerve biopsy is indicated in the diagnosis of treatable vasculitic conditions and if the disease being diagnosed is associated with neuropathic features; biopsy of the sural nerve is frequently carried out.[36]

As with muscle biopsies, there are many other tools used to establish the diagnosis of neurologic conditions without relying on a tissue sample, including nerve

Table 2 Routinely stained molecules and structures	
Stain	**Target Molecules/Structures**
Hematoxylin and eosin	Basophilic and eosinophilic cell structures
NADH	Mitochondria and endoplasmic reticulum
Fiber specific	Type 1 or 2 myofibers
Modified Gomori trichrome	Mitochondria
Periodic acid–Schiff	Polysaccharides including glycogen
Sudan black	Fats
Immunohistochemical stains	Specific to individual molecules
Immunofluorescence	Specific to individual molecules
Enzymatic reactions	Specific to individual enzymatic reactions/products

conduction velocity, electromyography, and autonomic and sensory studies. The analysis and description of these studies is beyond the scope of this article.

Nerve Biopsy Technique

As with muscle biopsy, a biopsy of the symptomatic nerve should be taken; sometimes this is a sensory nerve, other times a motor nerve. In the case of a sensory nerve, a segment can be resected and the patient might have recovery of some sensory function. For motor nerve biopsies, each nerve bundle is tested with electric stimulation to see if it has motor function; the bundle that does not cause muscle contraction is resected. As with a sensory nerve biopsy, there might be some sensory loss that resolves with time.

The biopsy of the sural nerve is explained here. The sural nerve is an easily accessible peripheral nerve commonly associated with sensory neuropathies. Its natural course is between the lateral malleolus and the Achilles tendon. The lesser saphenous vein also courses just lateral to the sural nerve and compression along the proximal leg will cause the vein to distend. After the landmarks are identified, the region is infiltrated with a local anesthetic. Next, a 2- to 3-cm incision is made between the fibula and the Achilles tendon. The subcutaneous tissue is then dissected bluntly and sharply. Care is taken to avoid damaging the nerve and therefore bipolar cautery is used instead of monopolar cautery due to decreased likelihood of thermal injury. The nerve is dissected away from the lesser saphenous vein in a careful manner.[36]

If diffuse neuropathy is suspected a fasicular nerve biopsy should be taken; in the case of neuropathy of a patchy distribution, a whole nerve biopsy is needed. The biopsy specimen is attached to a small gauge needle and suspended in fixative. Care must be taken to avoid physical manipulation of the nerve and the needle suspension prevents the nerve from contracting/coiling.[36]

The skin is then closed in the usual two-layered closure with a deep dermal absorbable suture and a mattressed nonabsorbable skin suture.

Nerve Biopsy Complications

The most common complications of a peripheral sensory nerve biopsy are allodynia, anesthesia, and paresthesias. These are seemingly related to the length of the nerve resection and will resolve over time (most within the first 18 months postsurgery). The degree of systemic neuropathic disease, such as diabetes mellitus, will correspond to the duration of neuropathic pain.

Other complications of nerve biopsies include local wound issues such as infection and wound breakdown, which occur less than 20% of the time.[36]

Discussion

Muscle and nerve biopsies are used for the diagnosis of a variety of medical problems. Although there are other genetic and biochemical markers now available that can diagnose diseases previously proven by biopsy, these surgical techniques still have appropriate uses. Although the procedures are straightforward, there are important technical issues to assist in getting the best specimen to avoid confounding disease diagnosis.

REFERENCES

1. Hansen SL. Skin and Subcutaneous tissue. In: Brunicardi FC, editor. Schwartz's principles of surgery. 8th edition. New York: McGraw-Hill Professional; 2004. p. 437.

2. Zuber TJ. Minimal excision technique for epidermoid (sebaceous) cysts. Am Fam Physician 2002;65(7):1409–12, 1417–8, 1420.

3. Moore RB, Fagan EB, Hulkower S, et al. Clinical inquiries. What's the best treatment for sebaceous cysts? J Fam Pract 2007;56(4):315–6.

4. Chandawarkar RY, Rodriquez P, Roussalis J, et al. Minimal-scar segmental extraction of lipomas: study of 122 consecutive procedures. Dermatol Surg 2005;31(1):59–63 [discussion: 63–4].

5. Brenn T. Neoplasms of Subcutaneous Fat. In: Wolff K, Goldsmith LA, Katz SI, et al, editors. Fitzpatrick's dermatology in general medicine. 7th edition. New York: McGraw-Hill; 2008. p. 1164–5, 90–3.

6. Kransdorf MJ, Bancroft LW, Peterson JJ, et al. Imaging of fatty tumors: distinction of lipoma and well-differentiated liposarcoma. Radiology 2002;224(1):99–104.

7. Gaskin CM, Helms CA. Lipomas, lipoma variants, and well-differentiated liposarcomas (atypical lipomas): results of MRI evaluations of 126 consecutive fatty masses. AJR Am J Roentgenol 2004;182(3):733–9.

8. Serpell JW, Chen RY. Review of large deep lipomatous tumours. ANZ J Surg 2007;77(7):524–9.

9. Salam GA. Lipoma excision. Am Fam Physician 2002;65(5):901–4.

10. Al-Qattan MM, Al-Lazzam AM, Al Thunayan A, et al. Classification of benign fatty tumours of the upper limb. Hand Surg 2005;10(1):43–59.

11. Kumar V. Robbins & Cotran pathologic basis of disease. 7th edition. Philadelphia: Saunders; 2004. p. 782–4.

12. Brennan M, Singer S. Sarcomas of the Soft Tissue and Bone. In: DeVita VT, editor. DeVita, Hellman, Rosenberg's cancer: principles & practice of oncology. 8th edition. Philadelphia: Lippincott Williams & Wilkins; 2008. p. 1750–2.

13. Yong M, Raza AS, Greaves TS, et al. Fine-needle aspiration of a pleomorphic lipoma of the head and neck: a case report. Diagn Cytopathol 2005;32(2):110–3.

14. Johnson RA. Benign Neoplasms and Hyperplasias. Subsection: Miscellaneous cysts and pseudocysts; Subsection: Benign dermal and subcutaneous neoplasms and hyperplasias. In: Fitzpatrick T, editor. Fitzpatrick's color atlas and synopsis of clinical dermatology. New York: McGraw-Hill; 2005.

15. Rotunda AM, Ablon G, Kolodney MS. Lipomas treated with subcutaneous deoxycholate injections. J Am Acad Dermatol 2005;53(6):973–8.

16. Campen R, Mankin H, Louis DN, et al. Familial occurrence of adiposis dolorosa. J Am Acad Dermatol 2001;44(1):132–6.

17. Uglesic V, Knezevic P, Milic M, et al. Madelung syndrome (benign lipomatosis): clinical course and treatment. Scand J Plast Reconstr Surg Hand Surg 2004;38(4):240–3.

18. Waite KA, Eng C. Protean PTEN: form and function. Am J Hum Genet 2002;70(4):829–44.

19. Herrmann SM, Adler YD, Schmidt-Petersen K, et al. The concomitant occurrence of multiple epidermal cysts, osteomas and thyroid gland nodules is not diagnostic for Gardner syndrome in the absence of intestinal polyposis: a clinical and genetic report. Br J Dermatol 2003;149(4):877–83.

20. Buisson P, Leclair MD, Jacquemont S, et al. Cutaneous lipoma in children: 5 cases with Bannayan-Riley-Ruvalcaba syndrome. J Pediatr Surg 2006;41(9):1601–3.

21. Genuardi M, Klutz M, Devriendt K, et al. Multiple lipomas linked to an RB1 gene mutation in a large pedigree with low penetrance retinoblastoma. Eur J Hum Genet 2001;9(9):690–4.

22. Erkek E, Hizel S, Sanly C, et al. Clinical and histopathological findings in Bannayan-Riley-Ruvalcaba syndrome. J Am Acad Dermatol 2005;53(4):639–43.

23. Finkelstein SE. Skin and Soft Tissue Tumors. In: Klingensmith ME, editor. Washington manual of surgery. 5th edition. Philadelphia: Lippincott Williams & Wilkins; 2007. p. 431–2.

24. Leppard BJ. Epidermoid cysts and polyposis coli. Proc R Soc Med 1974;67(10): 1036–7.

25. Goldstein BG. Benign neoplasms of the skin. Waltham, MA: UpToDate; 2008.

26. Lee HE, Yang CH, Chen CH, et al. Comparison of the surgical outcomes of punch incision and elliptical excision in treating epidermal inclusion cysts: a prospective, randomized study. Dermatol Surg 2006;32(4):520–5.

27. Dolsky RL. Surgical removal of lipoma by lipo-suction surgery. Am J Cosmet Surg 1986;3:27.

28. Choi CW, Kim BJ, Moon SE, et al. Treatment of lipomas assisted with tumescent liposuction. J Eur Acad Dermatol Venereol 2007;21(2):243–6.

29. Kitamura K, Takahashi T, Yamaguchi T, et al. Primary resection of infectious epidermal cyst. J Am Coll Surg 1994;179(5):607.

30. Sempowski IP. Sebaceous cysts. Ten tips for easier excision. Can Fam Physician 2006;52:315–7.

31. Andrews K, Ghavami A, Mowlavi A, et al. The youthful forehead: placement of skin incisions in hidden furrows. Dermatol Surg 2000;26(5):489–90.

32. Satyaprakash AK, Sheehan DJ, Sangueza OP. Proliferating trichilemmal tumors: a review of the literature. Dermatol Surg 2007;33(9):1102–8.

33. Wade CL, Haley JC, Hood AF. The utility of submitting epidermoid cysts for histologic examination. Int J Dermatol 2000;39(4):314–5.

34. Bennett DL, Groves M, Blake J, et al. The use of nerve and muscle biopsy in the diagnosis of vasculitis: a 5 year retrospective study. J Neurol Neurosurg Psychiatr 2008;79(12):1376–81.

35. Seidman RJ. Muscle biopsy and the pathology of skeletal muscle. Omaha, NE: e-Medicine; 2006.

36. Bevilacqua NJ, et al. Technique of the sural nerve biopsy. J Foot Ankle Surg 2007; 46(2):139–42.

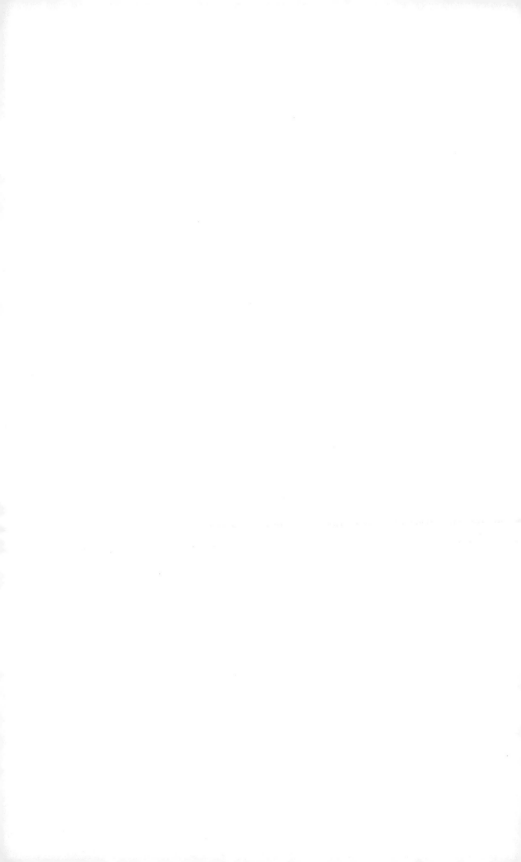

Pilonidal Disease and Hidradenitis

Alfonso L. Velasco, MD[a,b,]*, Wade W. Dunlap, MD[c]

KEYWORDS

- Pilonidal disease • Pilonidal sinus • Surgical treatment
- Procedure • Hidradenitis suppurativa • Sacrococcygeal

PILONIDAL DISEASE

Pilonidal disease is a common problem that affects young adults. Its clinical presentation ranges from a simple intergluteal skin pit with minimal symptoms to a complex infection in the subcutaneous tissues of the sacral area with multiple sinuses and a secondary opening. The surgical management of pilonidal disease should be tailored to the individual clinical presentation and its goal is the resolution of pilonidal disease with low recurrence and low morbidity. This article reviews the epidemiology, etiology, clinical presentation, and surgical treatment of pilonidal disease with emphasis on the selection of the appropriate procedure according to the presenting clinical problem.

Epidemiology

Pilonidal disease is most frequently seen in young adults. It is rarely seen after the age of 45 years. Its incidence is not known, but by some estimates it affects up to 0.7% of adolescents and young adults.[1] In a report from a British Hospital it accounted for two annual admissions.[2] It affects men more frequently than women in a ratio of 3–4:1.

History and Pathogenesis

Pilonidal disease was first described by O. H. Mayo in 1833.[3] However, others believe that A. W. Anderson's letter to the editor in the *Boston Medical Surgical Journal* of 1847 represents the first description of pilonidal disease.[4] The term "pilonidal" (nest of hair) was coined by Hodges in 1880.[5] The etiology of pilonidal disease has been controversial. Initially the cause was believed to be embryologic with an inborn defect

[a] Department of General and Colorectal Surgery, Marshfield Clinic and Saint Joseph's Hospital, 1000 North Oak Avenue, Marshfield, WI 54449, USA
[b] Department of Surgery, H4/785 Clinical Science Center, University of Wisconsin School of Medicine and Public Health, 600 Highland Avenue, Madison, WI 53792, USA
[c] Department of Surgery, Marshfield Clinic and Saint Joseph's Hospital, 1000 North Oak Avenue, Marshfield, WI 54449, USA
* Corresponding author. Department of General and Colorectal Surgery, Marshfield Clinic and Saint Joseph's Hospital, 1000 North Oak Avenue, Marshfield, WI 54449.
E-mail address: velasco.alfonso@marshfieldclinic.org (A.L. Velasco).

Surg Clin N Am 89 (2009) 689–701
doi:10.1016/j.suc.2009.02.003
0039-6109/09/$ – see front matter © 2009 Elsevier Inc. All rights reserved.

surgical.theclinics.com

of the skin in the intergluteal region secondary to a remnant of the medullary canal and infolding of the surface epithelium. However, several lines of evidence point toward an acquired cause: (1) the disease does not present at birth, but in young adults; (2) it is more frequent in men of hirsute complexion; and (3) certain occupations predispose people to develop pilonidal disease. Examples include "jeep disease" described by Buie[6] occurring in young soldiers riding jeeps on rough roads, and the presentation of pilonidal-like disease in the interdigital spaces of hairdressers and sheep-shearers.[7,8] It is possible that both theories are correct.

Presently, the acquired theory is the most popular. The details of the acquired mechanism vary widely. Bascom[9] believes that hair follicles in the natal cleft become distended with keratin and then infected, forming an abscess. After the abscess is formed, hairs can enter though the skin pit of the hair follicle into the abscess cavity. Karydakis[10] proposes that hair with chisel-like roots inserts itself into the natal cleft leading to foreign body tissue reaction and infection.

Whatever the precise cause of pilonidal disease, its anatomic features are well established. They include a midline pit in the natal cleft (primary opening) that extends into a subcutaneous fibrous tract (pilonidal sinus) and a secondary opening, located off the midline, which is characterized by drainage of purulent or serosanguinous fluid, the presence of granulation tissue, and hypertrophy of the epithelium surrounding the opening. Occasionally, hair extrudes from the primary opening. The pilonidal sinus tract has a wide individual variation. Ninety-three percent run cephalad, they may be single or multiple, and they can be short or long leading to a variety of clinical presentations. If the pilonidal sinus runs caudad (7%) the secondary opening may resemble the opening of a fistula in ano. Pilonidal sinuses are lined with granulation tissue and contain foreign matter such as hair and epithelial debris.

Clinical Presentation and Diagnosis

In general, the diagnosis of pilonidal disease is straightforward on clinical grounds. Symptoms may vary from pain in the sacrococcygeal region to chronic drainage of purulent fluid from the same area. Frequently, patients will describe intermittent symptoms of pain and drainage followed by long quiescent periods. Physical examination confirms the diagnosis and the findings can be listed as follows:

Acute pilonidal abscess: This is characterized by a tender fluctuant subcutaneous mass and surrounding cellulitis located off the midline of the natal cleft in the sacrococcygeal region. The onset of symptoms is rapid and pain may be severe. Primary openings are frequently seen on the midline natal cleft.

Chronic pilonidal sinus: In these cases there is a primary opening on the midline of the natal cleft sometimes with extruding hair located 4 to 5 cm cephalad to the anus. There may be a secondary opening located off the midline. The secondary opening is usually cephalad to the primary opening and at a variable distance from it.

Complicated pilonidal sinuses: Findings may include multiple skin pits on the midline of the natal cleft that lead to multiple sinuses and a secondary opening at variable distances from the midline. Partially drained abscesses may also be present.

Recurrent pilonidal disease: Findings in this situation are variable and include the previous surgical scar with different degrees of surrounding fibrosis. The primary opening may or may not be visible and one or multiple secondary openings may be present.

The differential diagnosis of pilonidal disease includes skin furuncles, hidradenitis suppurativa, anal fistula, and osteomyelitis with draining sinuses. Less common differential diagnoses include actinomycosis and syphilitic or tuberculous granulomas.

Treatment

The goals of treatment of pilonidal disease are to provide cure with procedures that have low recurrence and morbidity, and facilitate rapid return to normal activity. The surgeon must tailor the magnitude of the procedure to the presenting clinical problem.

Pilonidal abscess

Drainage of a pilonidal abscess can be performed in the office or in the emergency room under local anesthesia. A longitudinal incision is made off the midline and the purulent fluid drained. The skin edges of the incision are trimmed making the pilonidal cavity an open wound. The hair around the wound is shaved and the wound is lightly packed with gauze. Patients are asked to keep the area clean, changing the dressing twice a day until the wound is closed. Once the wound has healed the recurrence rate of either an abscess or formation of a pilonidal sinus may be as high as 50%.

Pilonidal sinus

Depending on the complexity of the pilonidal sinus or sinuses, the treatment can be nonoperative or operative. Operations for pilonidal sinuses include incisional procedures, excisional procedures with or without primary closure, and excisional procedures with flap closure.

Nonoperative treatment

This approach has been advocated by some investigators. The principles of this treatment include shaving the area involved and strict hygiene of the natal cleft. Klass[11] reported on 15 patients undergoing nonoperative treatment. Eleven patients were cured with follow-up at 3 years.

Injection of phenol into the sinus tract has been described by Schnider and colleagues.[12] Forty-five patients were treated with 1 to 2 mL of 80% phenol. The injection was performed under local anesthesia. Only 60% of patients healed in an average of 6 weeks, and 11% of patients developed abscesses. The authors do not use nor recommend this treatment.

Incisional procedures

Incision with marsupialization With this technique, the entire sinus tract is opened from the primary to the secondary openings. Hair is removed and granulation tissue is thoroughly curetted. The fibrous tract is left in place and sutured to the edges of the skin, reducing the wound surface by 50% to 60% (**Fig. 1**). This procedure is simple and can be performed in the outpatient setting under local anesthesia and sedation. Soya and Rothemberger[13] reported on 125 patients in a retrospective study who had undergone this procedure. The length of follow-up is not clear, however, the recurrence rate was only 6% and the time to healing was 3 to 20 weeks (average 4 weeks). Two other studies have shown similar good results.[14,15]

Lateral incision and excision of midline pits In this technique, the midline pit or pits are excised. The approach to the sinus tract is through a longitudinal incision off the midline of the natal cleft. The sinus tract is then cleaned and curetted (**Fig. 2**). Bascom[16] studied 149 patients who had undergone this procedure. At a mean follow-up of 3.5 years, the cure rate was 84%.

Excisional procedures

Excision with or without closure En bloc excision is made of the entire pilonidal sinus down to the sacrococcygeal fascia. The wound is packed with moist gauze and dressings are changed daily. Sondenaa and colleagues[17] studied 153 patients who had undergone this procedure. Seventy-eight patients received pre-operative antibiotics

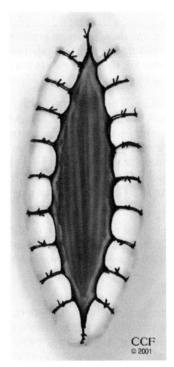

Fig.1. In marsupialization, the tracts are identified and unroofed. In this technique, excision (versus unroofing) of the tracts and pits can be done. The wound is curettaged. In an effort to decrease the size of the wound, and in turn accelerate wound healing, skin edges are sewn to the fibrotic base of the wound. (*Courtesy of* Cleveland Clinic Foundation, Inc., Cleveland, OH. Reprinted with the permission of The Cleveland Clinic Center for Medical Art & Photography © 2009. All Rights Reserved.)

and 75 patients did not receive antibiotics. The complication rate and wound healing was similar in the two groups. After 1 month, the rate of wound healing was 69% and the complication rate was 64% for the group who received antibiotics; for the group who did not receive antibiotics, the rate of wound healing was 44% and the complication rate was 43%. Kronborg and colleagues[18] obtained somewhat better results when they closed the wounds after en bloc excision.

In our opinion, en bloc excision of the pilonidal sinus carries a higher morbidity and no improvement in healing rate compared with the incisional procedure described earlier.

Excisional procedure with flap closure
Excision and Z-plasty This procedure is well suited for the treatment of the complex pilonidal sinus. To avoid the recurrence or breakdown of the midline wound, the pilonidal sinus is removed and then the natal cleft is obliterated with a Z-plasty, which effectively flattens the natal cleft. In this procedure the entire pilonidal sinus is removed, the limbs of the Z-plasty are fashioned at 30° angles from the wound axis. Full thickness subcutaneous skin flaps are raised and then transposed and sutured (**Fig. 3**). A suction drain is left in place to avoid formation of a seroma. Toubanakis[19] reported on 110 patients treated with Z-plasty. There were no recurrences in this series.

Although the reported results on excision and Z-plasty are good, the authors believe this surgery is too extensive for treatment of simple, uncomplicated pilonidal sinuses.

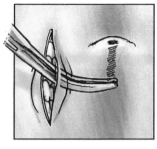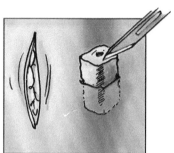

Fig. 2. In the Bascom operation, midline pilonidal pits or follicles are excised. One to ten follicles can be removed, leaving wounds 2 to 4 mm in diameter. The sinuses or cavity are opened through an incision 2 cm lateral and parallel to the natal cleft. The lateral incision undermines the midline and gauze is pushed through the cavity to "scrub out" hair and granulation tissue. (*Courtesy of* Cleveland Clinic Foundation, Inc., Cleveland, OH. Reprinted with the permission of The Cleveland Clinic Center for Medical Art & Photography © 2009. All Rights Reserved.)

Advancing flap operation (Karydakis procedure) The goal of this technique is to avoid a suture line on the midline of the natal cleft. The effectiveness of this technique is predicated on the belief that recurrences occur from hairs that are forced into the skin pits of the natal cleft and a midline suture line. Karydakis described a technique in which a "semilateral" incision is made around the pilonidal sinus all the way down to the presacral fascia (**Fig. 4**). Mobilization of the subcutaneous flap is performed on the side closer to the midline and then the flap is sutured to the opposite side effectively placing the suture line off the midline. A suction drain is left in place. In a large series of 7,471 patients undergoing the advancing flap procedure, the recurrence rate was 1% at 2 to 20 years of follow-up, and the complication rate was 8.5%.[10,20]

The Karydakis procedure is effective but frequently requires overnight admission to the hospital and is, perhaps, too large a procedure for the treatment of small, simple pilonidal cysts. However, it is an excellent procedure for the treatment of large, complex pilonidal sinuses.

Treatment of the Unhealed Pilonidal Wound

Regardless of the surgical procedure used in the primary treatment of pilonidal disease, a frequent postoperative problem is the unhealed wound. This complication seems to be less frequent if the suture line is placed off the midline natal cleft. The unhealed wound is characterized by the presence of abundant granulation tissue at its base. If the unhealed wound is small, treatment includes curettage, removal of hair surrounding the wound, and application of silver nitrate with strict local hygiene. For larger unhealed wounds, it is best to excise the wound and reconstruct the area with a flap procedure. Z-plasty, gluteus maximus myocutaneous flap (**Fig. 5**), and Bascom's Cleft Closure procedure (**Fig. 6**) are all effective for the treatment of large, unhealed wounds.

Summary

Pilonidal disease occurs frequently and affects primarily the young adult. Most patients require surgical treatment. Many surgical procedures are available. It is

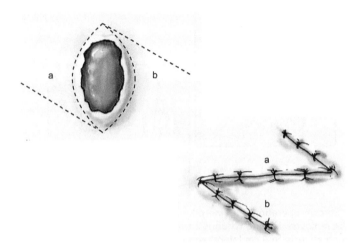

Fig. 3. Z-Plasty obliterates the natal cleft and provides increased transverse length by recruiting lateral tissue. The midline sinus is excised. Limbs of the Z are cut at the ends of the midline wound. Subcutaneous skin flaps are raised down to the level of the fascia and transposed as shown with the limb of the a and b flaps moved into place as shown. Finally the skin is closed. (*Courtesy of* Cleveland Clinic Foundation, Inc., Cleveland, OH. Reprinted with the permission of The Cleveland Clinic Center for Medical Art & Photography © 2009. All Rights Reserved.)

important to match the magnitude of the procedure to the complexity of pilonidal disease. For small, single pilonidal sinuses, incision and marsupialization may be the treatment of choice. For larger pilonidal sinuses excision of the midline pit with lateral incision and curettage of the sinus offers fast recovery and low morbidity. Wide excision with any of the flap reconstruction techniques should be reserved for complex or recurrent pilonidal sinuses, and for treatment of large unhealed wounds.

HIDRADENITIS SUPPURATIVA

Hidradenitis suppurativa (HS) is a disease of the skin. It affects primarily young individuals and its clinical course is characterized by chronicity with frequent flare-ups followed by quiescent periods. The severity of HS is variable. At one end of the

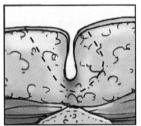
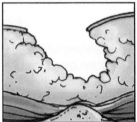
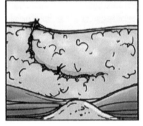

Fig. 4. Excision of the disease and primary closure is one surgical option. In an effort to improve on this technique, Karydakis modified the procedure. The midline sinus is excised elliptically and the wound closed lateral to the midline. To do this, a thick flap is created by undercutting the medial wound edge and advancing it across the midline. By doing this, the natal cleft is flattened and the entire suture line is positioned lateral to the midline. (*Courtesy of* Cleveland Clinic Foundation, Inc., Cleveland, OH. Reprinted with the permission of The Cleveland Clinic Center for Medical Art & Photography © 2009. All Rights Reserved.)

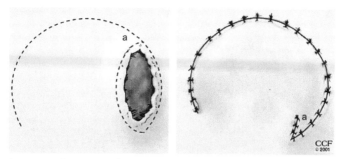

Fig. 5. The gluteus maximus musculocutaneous flap consists of the creation of a large rotational buttock flap. The procedure permits radical excision of all diseased tissue and fills the dead space with bulky, well-vascularized, and compliant tissue. Large defects can be covered using this approach. This procedure carries the highest degree of difficulty and potential morbidity of all approaches, and is used if other conventional procedures have failed. (*Courtesy of* Cleveland Clinic Foundation, Inc., Cleveland, OH. Reprinted with the permission of The Cleveland Clinic Center for Medical Art & Photography © 2009. All Rights Reserved.)

spectrum the disease may involve a small area of the skin causing minimal problems. At the other end HS may be a devastating disease causing serious disability. The areas of skin most frequently affected are the axilla, inframammary region, inguinal areas, and the perineal and perianal skin. The quality of life of those affected by HS may be significantly diminished because of the recalcitrant, painful lesions with malodorous discharge.[21,22]

Although HS is located in areas with a high concentration of apocrine glands, it seems that the inciting event is the occlusion of hair follicles and their subsequent dilation and rupture with spillage of keratin and bacteria into the dermis leading to the typical clinical presentation of HS. The realization that the main event in the causation of HS involves the hair follicle and not the apocrine glands has led to the suggestion of the term acne inversa.[23,24]

Many different forms of treatment have been advocated in the management of HS. They range from simple local measures of hygiene to wide surgical excision of affected areas. The treatment should be tailored to each individual patient and the authors would like to emphasize that patients with HS are better served by a multidisciplinary approach involving dermatologists, surgeons, a wound clinic, physical therapists and, on occasion, psychologists.

This review discusses the epidemiology, natural history, etiology, pathogenesis, clinical presentation, and treatment of HS, with emphasis on its surgical management.

Epidemiology and Natural History

The prevalence of HS has been estimated to be between 1 in 100[25] and 1 in 600[26] people. It is more common in women than men at a ratio of 2:5.[27] Perianal HS, however, is twice as frequent in men than women.[28] The most frequent age at presentation is between the second and third decades of life.[29]

HS is a chronic disease. In one study 90% of patients had had the disease for an average of 19 years.[30] HS is not relentlessly progressive, but characterized by periods of quiescence and activity. It seems that as patients become older the disease becomes less active.

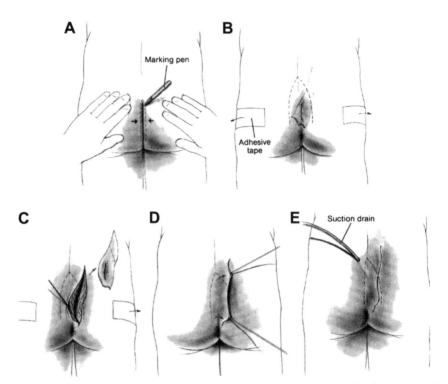

Fig. 6. (A) Natural lines of contact of the buttock cheeks are marked. (B) The buttock cheeks are taped apart. (C) The unhealed wound is excised in a triangular shape. (D) After the skin flap is raised out to the marked line, the tapes are released. The skin flap is positioned to overlap the edges of the wound on the opposite side. Excess skin is incised. A closed suction drain is placed in the subcutaneous tissue, which is closed with 3-0 chromic catgut. (E) The skin is closed with subcuticular 4-0 polydioxanone sutures. (*From* Fazio VW, editor. Current therapy in colon and rectal surgery. Toronto (ON): BC Decker, 1990. p. 32–9; with permission.)

Etiology

The underlying factor predisposing to occlusion of the hair follicles in areas affected by HS has not been elucidated. Several medical and nonmedical conditions have been associated with HS. A positive family history is present in 26% of patients.[25] An autosomal-dominant inheritance has been reported by Fitzsimmons and colleagues.[31,32] Endocrine factors may promote HS. However, the available scientific evidence is not sufficient to fully support this argument. HS is associated with acne vulgaris,[33] premenstrual flare-ups,[34] and the use of birth control pills,[35] which point to the possible promoting role of sex hormones. Barth and colleagues[36] studied 66 women with HS and none of them had evidence of hyperandrogenism.

Smoking is more frequent in patients with HS. In one study 70% of patients with perianal disease were smokers.[34] Obesity may be an aggravating rather than a causative factor in patients with HS.[37] Bacteriologic studies suggest that bacterial contamination and infection are secondary to follicular occlusion. A study of cultures obtained from early HS lesions demonstrated that half of the cultures were negative. *Staphylococcus aureus* and coagulase negative staphylococci were the organisms most frequently isolated.[38,39]

Pathogenesis

The initial step in the pathogenesis of HS, as determined by the study of pathologic specimens, is occlusion of the hair follicles.[23,24] Dilatation and rupture of hair follicles into the dermis leads to dermal infiltration by inflammatory cells, giant cells, and formation of sinus tracts and fibrosis.[22] Apocrine glands are compound sweat glands found in the axilla, genitofemoral, perineal and perianal areas, periareolar, inframammary, and periumbilical areas. Inflammation and destruction of these glands seems to be incidental rather than a causative factor of HS.[24]

Clinical Presentation and Diagnosis

Patients with HS complain of pain and malodorous discharge originating in the area of affected skin. Physical examination reveals indurated subcutaneous nodules, subcutaneous abscesses and draining skin sinuses that may coalesce forming a network of subcutaneous cavities and tracts with extensive fibrosis. Overall, the regions most frequently affected are the axillary, inguinal, and perineal regions.[40]

The diagnosis is based on clinical findings and diagnostic biopsies are seldom necessary. However, if the differential diagnosis includes perianal Crohn disease or cancer, biopsies should be obtained to establish a definitive diagnosis. Other differential diagnoses include skin carbuncle, dermoid cysts, furuncles, granuloma inguinale, pilonidal cysts, skin tuberculosis, perianal cryptoglandular fistulas, and perianal Crohn disease. Gower-Rousseu and colleagues[41] described the association of Crohn disease and HS in two families. However, it is not clear if this association is circumstantial or significant.

As described earlier, the clinical presentation of HS encompasses a wide spectrum of severity. This fact and the chronicity and relapsing nature of the disease mandate the formulation of tailored individual treatment plans delivered by a multidisciplinary team.

Treatment

Once the diagnosis of HS is made, an assessment of its severity and location allows different treatment modalities to be used according to the individual situation. One or multiple forms of treatment may apply to a single patient. The different treatment modalities are reviewed separately.

Nonsurgical treatment

Personal considerations First, the patient should be educated about the chronic and relapsing nature of HS. They should also know that the disease is not contagious or due to poor hygiene.[42]

General measures Avoiding skin irritants (shaving, depilation, and deodorants), tight clothing, prolonged heat exposure, losing weight, and smoking cessation are initiatives that make sense, but their efficacy is only anecdotal.

Antibiotic treatment Topical clindamycin[43] and oral administration of tetracycline[44] are effective at controlling local inflammation in areas affected by HS. However, short-term antibiotic therapy does not alter the natural history of HS, which frequently relapses after discontinuation of treatment. Long-term suppressive antibiotic therapy has been suggested in the treatment of severe recurrent disease.[42] It is unclear if long-term therapy prevents progression or changes the natural history of HS.

Hormonal therapy The role of sex hormones has not been clearly established in HS. Given the indirect evidence of hormones promoting HS, several investigators have attempted to define the effectiveness of antihormonal therapy. Mortimer and colleagues,[45] in a randomized controlled trial, found decreased disease activity in patients treated with the antiandrogen, cyproterone acetate. In another study, finasteride, used in the treatment of benign prostatic hypertrophy, improved HS in two patients.[46] Isoretinoin (Accutane), a derivative of vitamin A, reduces epithelial differentiation and sebaceous secretions. Its use in the treatment of acne has been well established. However, the results in the treatment of HS have been less favorable. Presently, isoretinoin at a dose of 0.5 to 1.0 mg/kg daily may be used to decrease inflammation in areas of HS before surgical excision.[47] Acitretin, used to treat psoriasis, may be effective for HS at a dose of 25 mg twice daily.[48] Retinoids are teratogenic and must be avoided during pregnancy.

Immunosuppression Cyclosporine[49] and infliximab[50] may ameliorate inflammation in severe HS. Given the toxicity, side effects and lack of clinical studies defining their therapeutic role, immunosuppressive therapy cannot be recommended for routine use in HS.

Surgical treatment
The surgical management of HS may be divided into two categories: surgery to control local infection and surgery performed with curative intent.

Surgery to control local infection Patients with HS may present with a subcutaneous abscess. These patients are treated with incision and drainage of the abscess. Then, depending on the individual circumstances, the patient is allocated to one of the multiple forms of nonsurgical management or to further surgery with curative intent once local inflammatory changes subside. On occasion, patients may present with an infected sinus tract and surrounding cellulitis. These patients may benefit from unroofing and marsupialization of the tract and subsequent allocation to other forms of therapy if needed.

Surgery with curative intent It is well established that, to prevent recurrence, the entire affected area must be removed. In some patients, the area of skin involved is so large that complete excision is not advisable. The location of HS (perianal or perineal) may also prevent complete excision.

Pre-operatively, attempts at decreasing local inflammation with antibiotics or retinoids[47] may improve postoperative healing and prevent complications.

Once the area with HS has been removed, the resulting wound may be approached in different ways. If the wound is small, it can be closed primarily without tension. Greely[51] and Paletta[52] reported decreased morbidity, length of hospitalization, and postoperative disability if primary closure is used. For larger wounds, the defect may be left open to close by secondary intention.[53] In these cases, active participation of wound specialists is invaluable. Regular dressing changes are important to keep the wound clean and avoid infection. In many cases physiotherapy is started early to prevent disabling contractures. Shahzad and colleagues reported 3 cases of advanced HS. All three underwent wide local excision and the wounds were left to heal by secondary intention. Two of their patients required physiotherapy to treat contractures. All patients tolerated the procedure well and had no recurrences.[53]

Perineal and perianal wounds are treated by allowing the wound to heal by secondary intention. A colostomy is rarely necessary after excision of perianal HS.

Large wounds may also be treated by immediate or delayed split thickness skin grafting. Blackburn and colleagues[54] described the use of negative pressure dressings to bolster skin grafts. Negative pressure dressings are particularly attractive if dealing with large contour wounds.

The use of local or distant flaps is not routinely advocated in HS. Flaps may be used in cases of complex wounds or in the surgical treatment of skin contractures.

The authors believe the procedure of choice in most patients with HS is complete excision followed by wound closure by secondary intention. The wound clinic is an active participant in the care of these patients. The recurrence rate after wide surgical excision has been reported at 0% for perianal disease, 3% for axillary disease and 37% for inguinoperineal disease. Radiotherapy[55] and laser treatment[56] have been used to treat HS. However, the results of these treatments do not compare favorably with wide surgical excision.

Summary

HS is a skin disease that affects young adults. It is a chronic condition with intermittent flare-ups and periods of quiescence. Its severity is variable and can be characterized by minor, localized symptoms to severe debilitating disease. There is also a wide range of treatments. Treatment needs to be individualized for the clinical presentation and should involve a multidisciplinary team. If conservative measures fail and surgery is required, wide local excision with wound healing by secondary intention is the best form of therapy. Other surgical options are available and should be employed appropriately according to the individual clinical presentation.

REFERENCES

1. Rakinic J. Modern management of pilonidal disease. In: Cameron JL, editor. Current surgical therapy. Saint Louis (MO): Mosby; 2007. p. 299–305.
2. Chintapatla S, Safarani N, Kumar S, et al. Sacrococcygeal pilonidal sinus: historical review, pathologic insight and surgical options. Tech Coloproctol 2003;7:3–8.
3. Mayo OH. Observations on injuries and diseases of the rectum. London: Burgess and Hill; 1833. 45–6.
4. Anderson AW. Hair extracted from an ulcer [letter]. Boston Med Surg J 1847;36:74.
5. Hodges RM. Pilo-nidal sinus. Boston Med Surg J 1880;103:485–6.
6. Buie LA. Jeep disease (pilonidal disease of mechanized warfare). South Med J 1944;37:103–9.
7. Patel MR, Bassini L, Nashad R, et al. Barber's interdigital pilonidal sinus of the hand: a foreign body hair granuloma. J Hand Surg 1990;15A:652–5.
8. Phillips PJ. Web space sinus in a shearer. Med J Aust 1966;2:1152–3.
9. Bascom J. Pilonidal disease: origin from follicles of hairs and results of follicle removal as treatment. Surgery 1980;87:567–72.
10. Karydakis GE. Easy and successful treatment of pilonidal sinus after explanation of its causative process. Aust N Z J Surg 1992;62(5):385–9.
11. Klass AA. The so-called pilonidal sinus. Can Med Assoc J 1956;75:737–42.
12. Schneider IHF, Thaler K, Kockerling RF. Treatment of pilonidal sinuses by phenol injections. Int J Colorectal Dis 1994;9:200–2.
13. Solla JA, Rothenberger DA. Chronic pilonidal disease: an assessment of 150 cases. Dis Colon Rectum 1990;33:758–61.
14. Spivak H, Brooks VL, Nussbaum M, et al. Treatment of chronic pilonidal disease. Dis Colon Rectum 1996;39(10):1136–9.
15. Vaula JL, Badaro JA, Nacusse E, et al. Enformedad pilonidal sacrococcigea. Prensa Med Argent 1986;73:489–91.
16. Bascom J. Pilonidal disease: long-term results of follicle removal. Dis Colon Rectum 1983;26(12):800–7.

17. Sondenaa K, Nesvik I, Gullaksen FP, et al. The role of cefoxitin prophylaxis in chronic pilonidal sinus treated with excision and primary suture. J Am Coll Surg 1995;180(2):157–60.
18. Kronborg O, Christensen K, Zimmermann-Nielsen C. Chronic pilonidal disease: a randomized trial with a complete 3-year follow-up. Br J Surg 1985;72(4):303–4.
19. Toubanakis G. Treatment of pilonidal sinus disease with Z-plasty procedure (modified). Am Surg 1986;52:611–2.
20. Kitchen PR. Pilonidal sinus: experience with the Karydakis flap. Br J Surg 1996; 83(10):1452–5.
21. Jemec GBE. What's new in hidradenitis suppurativa? J Eur Acad Dermatol Venereol 2000;14:340–1.
22. Slade DEM, Powell BW, Mortimer PS. Hidradenitis suppurativa: pathogenesis and management. Br J Plast Surg 2003;56:451–61.
23. Plewig G, Steger M. Acne inversa (alias acne triad, acne tetrad or hidradenitis suppurativa). In: Marks R, Plewig G, editors. Acne and related disorders. London: Martin Dunitz; 1991. p. 345–57.
24. Jansen T, Plewig G. What's new in acne inversa (alias hidradenitis suppurativa)? J Eur Acad Dermatol Venereol 2000;14:342–3.
25. Jemec GBE, Heidenheim M, Nielsen NH. The prevalence of hidradenitis suppurativa and its potential precursor lesions. J Am Acad Dermatol 1996;35:191–4.
26. Harrison BJ, Mudge M, Hughes LE. The prevalence of hidradenitis suppurativa in South Wales. In: Marks R, Plewig G, editors. Acne and related disorders. London: Martin Dunitz; 1989. p. 365–6.
27. Wiseman MC. Hidradenitis suppurativa: a review. Dermatol Ther 2004;17:50–4.
28. Brown SC, Kazzazi N, Lord PH. Surgical treatment of perineal hidradenitis suppurativa with special reference to recognition of the perianal form. Br J Surg 1986; 73:978–80.
29. Parks RW, Parks TG. Pathogenesis, clinical features and management of hidradenitis suppurativa. Ann R Coll Surg Engl 1997;79:83–9.
30. von der Worth JM, Williams HC. The natural history of hidradenitis suppurativa. J Eur Acad Dermatol Venereol 2000;14:389–92.
31. Fitzsimmons JS, Guilbert PR, Fitzsimmons EM. Evidence of genetic factors in hidradenitis suppurativa. Br J Dermatol 1985;113:1–8.
32. Fitzsimmons JS, Fitzsimmons EM, Bilbert G. Familial hidradenitis suppurativa: evidence in favour of single gene transmission. J Med Genet 1984;21:281–5.
33. Mortimer PS, Dawber RPR, Gales M, et al. Mediation of hidradenitis suppurativa by androgens. BMJ 1986;292:245–8.
34. Wiltz O, Schoetz DJ, Murray JJ, et al. Perianal hidradenitis suppurativa: the Lahey clinic experience. Dis Colon Rectum 1990;33:731–4.
35. Stellon AG, Wakeling M. Hidradenitis suppurativa associated with use of oral contraceptives. BMJ 1989;298:28–9.
36. Barth JH, Layton AM, Cunliffe WJ. Endocrine factors in pre- and postmenstrual women with hidradenitis suppurativa. Br J Dermatol 1996;134:1057–9.
37. Jemec GBE. Body weight in hidradenitis suppurativa. In: Marks R, Plewig G, editors. Acne and related disorders. London: Martin Dunitz; 1989. p. 375–6.
38. Jemec GBE, Faber M, Gutschick E, et al. The bacteriology of hidradenitis suppurativa. Dermatology 1996;193:203–6.
39. Lapins J, Jarstrand C, Emtestam L. Coagulase-negative staphylococci are the most common bacteria found in cultures from the deep portions of hidradenitis suppurativa lesions, as obtained by carbon dioxide laser surgery. Br J Dermatol 1999;140:90–5.

40. Harrison BJ, Kumar S, Read GF, et al. Hidradenitis suppurativa: evidence for an endocrine abnormality. Br J Surg 1985;72:1002–4.
41. Gower-Rousseau C, Maunoury V, Colombel JF, et al. Hidradenitis suppurativa and Crohn's disease in two families: a significant association? [letter]. Am J Gastroenterol 1992;87:928.
42. Shah N. Hidradenitis suppurativa: a treatment challenge. Am Fam Physician 2005;72:1547–52.
43. Clemmensen OJ. Topical treatment of hidradenitis suppurativa with clindamycin. Int J Dermatol 1983;22:325–8.
44. Jemec GBE. The symptomatology of hidradenitis suppurativa in women. Br J Dermatol 1988;119:345–50.
45. Mortimer PS, Dawber RPR, Gales MA, et al. A double-blind cross-over trial of cyproterone acetate in females with hidradenitis suppurativa. Br J Dermatol 1986;115:263–8.
46. Farrell AM, Randall VA, Vafaee T, et al. Finasteride as a therapy for hidradenitis suppurativa. [letter]. Br J Dermatol 1999;141:1138–9.
47. Jansen T, Plewig G. Acne inversa. Int J Dermatol 1998;37:96–100.
48. Chow ETY, Mortimer PS. Successful treatment of hidradenitis suppurativa and retroauricular acne with etretinate. Br J Dermatol 1992;126:415.
49. Buckley DA, Rogers S. Cyclosporin-responsive hidradenitis suppurativa. J R Soc Med 1995;88:289–90.
50. Sullivan TP, Welsh E, Kerdel FA, et al. Infliximab for hidradenitis suppurativa. Br J Dermatol 2003;149:1046–9.
51. Greeley PW. Plastic surgical treatment of chronic suppurative hidradenitis. Plast Reconstr Surg 1951;7:143–6.
52. Paletta FX. Hidradenitis suppurativa: a pathologic study and the use of skin flaps. Plast Reconstr Surg 1963;31:307–15.
53. Ather S, Chan DSY, Leaper DJ, et al. Surgical treatment of hidradenitis suppurativa: case series and review of the literature. Int Wound J 2006;3:159–69.
54. Blackburn JH, Boemi L, Hall WW, et al. Negative-pressure dressings as a bolster for skin grafts. Ann Plast Surg 1998;40:453–7.
55. Frohlich D, Baaske D, Glatzel M. Radiotherapy of hidradenitis suppurativa – still valid today? Strahlenther Onkol 2000;176:286–9.
56. Laplins J, Sartorius K, Emtestam L. Scanner-assisted carbon dioxide laser surgery: a retrospective follow-up study of patients with hidradenitis suppurativa. J Am Acad Dermatol 2002;47:280–5.

Common Skin Cancers and Their Precursors

Alisha Arora, MD[b], John Attwood, MD[a],*

KEYWORDS

- Basil cell carcinoma • Squamous cell carcinoma
- Malignant melanoma • Precursor lesions

Skin is the largest organ in the body. Its functions include mechanical protection from the outside world, thermoregulation, sensation, fluid management, immunologic surveillance, and ultraviolet (UV) protection. Failure in the last regard leads to a spectrum of skin lesions, varying from benign precursors to skin cancer to outright malignancy. Skin cancers can be broadly categorized into two groups: nonmelanoma and melanoma. Nonmelanoma skin cancers are the most common cancers in the United States. More than 1,000,000 were diagnosed in 2008.[1] They are typically a disease of fair-skinned people lacking in melanin and correlate closely with sun exposure. As one would expect, these cancers increase in frequency with decreasing latitude (ie, greater sun exposure), outdoor occupation (ie, farmers), and increasing age. Skin cancers can be difficult to diagnose, because their appearances vary so widely in color, morphology, and texture. Likewise, the biologic potential can vary from indolence to aggressive morbidity and mortality. Melanoma occurs in all ethnic groups, although again an association with increased sun exposure and decreased melanin content is seen.[2]

RISK FACTORS IN CARCINOGENESIS

Skin cancer results from multifactorial causes, and these can be broadly divided into environmental and host factors. Environmental factors include exposure to UV radiation and ionizing radiation as well as chemical exposure (arsenic, polyaromatic hydrocarbons). Host factors include (HIV, human papillomavirus [HPV], transplant immunosuppression), genetic syndromes, and existence of precursor lesions. Within both of these subgroups, individual factors can be considered to be modifiable or fixed. By targeting the modifiable risk factors, it may be possible to reduce one's own lifetime risk of skin cancer.

UV radiation sits in the middle of the electromagnetic spectrum. Three groups exist: UVA (400–315 nm), UVB (315–290), and UVC (290–200 nm). Visible light is the 400 to 700 nm range. Only UVA and UVB rays penetrate the ozone stratosphere to reach the earth's surface; greater than 95% of that is in the UVA spectrum. Most sunscreens target these rays; however, the UVB rays produce the most carcinogenic effects on

[a] Plastic and Hand Surgical Associates, 244 Western Avenue, South Portland, ME 04106, USA
[b] Department of Plastic Surgery, Lahey Clinic, 41 Mall Road, Burlington, MA 01805, USA
* Corresponding author.
E-mail address: jattwood@plasticandhand.com (J. Attwood).

Surg Clin N Am 89 (2009) 703–712
doi:10.1016/j.suc.2009.03.007
0039-6109/09/$ – see front matter © 2009 Elsevier Inc. All rights reserved.
surgical.theclinics.com

skin cells. They directly injure DNA as well as DNA repair mechanisms and suppress cell-mediated immunity. UVA rays are thought to potentiate the damage of UVB. The UVA exposure from a tanning bed is greater that that given off by natural sunlight, so although UVB exposure is not a risk, caution and vigilance must still be exercised if suspicious lesions are seen in patients who choose to use tanning beds. Regular glass blocks UVB but screens out only 50% of UVA radiation. Cloud cover protects only from UV radiation by 20% to 40%, which is why it is recommended to wear sunscreen while outdoors even on cloudy days. Regular clothing provides little UV protection. Sunscreen provides a chemical or physical barrier to UV radiation if applied properly. About 2 mg/cm^2 of skin surface area constitutes an adequate dose and must be reapplied frequently to ensure coverage. Chemical sunscreens such as para-amninobenzoic acid derivatives, benzophenone, and cinnamates absorb UV radiation, both UVA and UVB, in today's broad-spectrum formulations. Physical sunscreens reduce UV exposure by reflecting the radiation and are the most effective. These products include zinc oxide and titanium dioxide.[3]

SQUAMOUS CELL CANCER
SCC Epidemiology

Squamous cell cancer (SCC) is the second most common skin cancer in the United States, preceded only by basal cell cancer (BCC).[4] It is 2 to 3 times more common in men than in women. The risk of developing SCC of the skin is proportional to the extent of sun exposure and, therefore, increases with age and decreases with distance from the equator. These tumors, although only one-fourth as prevalent as BCC, show a much stronger correlation with actinic damage than BCC. As one would expect then, lighter-skinned individuals with red or blond hair and blue or green eyes are more susceptible to developing SCC than are more pigmented individuals. Patients with xeroderma pigmentosum, an autosomal recessive defect in DNA repair mechanism, also develop both SCC and malignant melanoma as a result of UV-induced DNA damage. Actinic keratosis (AK) is the typical precursor lesion as well as radiation keratosis, leukoplakia, chronic ulcers and sinus tracts, scars, and areas of dermatitis. Bowen's disease of the skin is considered to be SCC in situ. HPV infection can also lead to SCC.[5]

Like BCC, SCC arises more commonly in the areas of the body most exposed to sunlight: Approximately 70% occur on the head and neck. Unlike BCC, SCC can also arise in old scars, typically burn scars, or in areas of chronic inflammation, such as sinus tracts. SCC arising in radiation fields, sites of chronic inflammation, or in immunosuppressed patients has a higher likelihood of metastasis than those that arise as a consequence of actinic damage. Lesions of the lip and ear also tend to be more aggressive. Overall, SCC tumors are faster growing than BCC.

AK is a precursor lesion to SCC and is considered by some to be SCC in situ. These lesions appear at the very least to reside on a continuum of cellular atypia. They are very common in sun-exposed areas of the body as a result of damage from UVB radiation. They present as red, pink, or brown scaly, erythematous plaques. The natural history of these lesions is thought to be either to regress spontaneously, persist, or to progress to invasive SCC. The true incidence and history are difficult to precisely describe as these lesions are likely to escape attention, and if treated, they receive repetitive, office-based, nonsurgical therapy that escapes national registries.

Histopathology

SCCs arise from the basal layer of epidermis. Rarely do they develop directly from normal skin; rather, they arise in association with an area of preexisting skin damage.

UV-induced alterations to the p53 tumor suppression gene pathway appear to be the primary insult allowing clonal expansion of malignant cells. Other genetic mutations may also contribute to the development of SCC.

Tumor grade is determined by the degree of cellular differentiation based on the ratio of atypical cells to normal epithelium. As in the case of melanoma, mitotic figures also determine the grade of the tumor. Other variables influencing tumor grade are cell size and shape, hyperchromasia, and keratinization. As one would expect, the higher the tumor grade (ie, the more aggressive the tumor), the less differentiated the cells are and the more prominent the mitotic figures are. Immunohistochemical staining may be necessary to differentiate high-grade SCC from DM. Epidermal cytokeratin antibody is specific for squamous epithelium, whereas S-100 protein antibody stains specifically for melanocytes and Langerhans cells.

Diagnosis

SCCs typically present as enlarging bumps that may have an irregular or reddened surface. The classic appearance is of a shallow ulcer with "heaped up" edges. They are typically more indurated and inflamed than BCC and often crust or ooze. This appearance is not to be confused with the "rodent ulcer," a type of BCC that is slow growing and eventually ulcerates but is only locally, not systemically, invasive. The term "Marjolin's ulcer" is used to describe epidermoid carcinomas that arise in chronically nonhealing tissues, typically in burns.

Clinical evidence of cranial nerve dysfunction, particularly in the facial trigeminal distribution, is an ominous sign of possible perineural invasion that indicates an aggressive tumor likely to recur. History of numbness, pain, or facial weakness or asymmetry should be carefully recorded as should size and location of the tumor.[6]

Suspicious lesions should be biopsied. Shave or incisional biopsy techniques are adequate; unlike melanoma, staging will not be affected by obscuring lesion depth. Reexcision is strongly recommended for positive specimens because of the high likelihood of residual microscopic tumor even if the biopsy site subsequently appears healed and free of tumor. Vigilance of biopsy is particularly important in old burn wounds, chronic nonhealing wounds, and scars that undergo acute changes to monitor for malignant transformation (Marjolin's ulcer).

Treatment

Treatment of SCC is based on many factors, not just tumor grade. Besides size and location of the tumor, one must take into consideration the overall health of the patients and their preference for treatment and cosmesis.

The American Academy of Dermatology has divided tumors into three groups based on depth. Lesions less than 4 mm deep are suitable for local excision. Lesions 4 to 8 mm deep should undergo surgical excision. Lesions greater than 8 mm likely deserve multimodality treatment with surgical excision, radiation, and possibly chemotherapy. Proposed margins for low-risk tumors of low grade and less than 2 cm are 4 mm; this extends to 6 mm for higher-risk neoplasms of higher grade and greater than 2 cm. It was found in one study that for lesions with a diameter less than 2 cm removed by Mohs microsurgery technique, 4 mm margins were sufficient to give a 98% complete excision rate for BCC and 100% excision rate for SCC.

Incomplete excision rates range in the literature from 5.8% to 15.9% with a 5-year likelihood of recurrence ranging from 5.7% to 8.1%. Negative margins should be ensured by frozen section before closure of the wound. Incomplete excision is associated with lesions of the ear and lesions presenting for reexcision. Recurrence is associated with lesions larger than 2 cm, lesions deeper than Clark's level four or five (invading the reticular dermis and subcutaneous tissues), depth greater than 4 mm, poor tumor histology, non–sun-exposed sites, immunosuppressed patients, and sites such as the ear or lip.[7]

Mohs micrographic technique was developed by Dr. Frederic E. Mohs in the 1930s to remove cutaneous malignancies 1 layer at a time and perform immediate pathologic analysis on either fixed or fresh tissue.[8] This meticulous technique is excellent for the face, ears, and other locations where preservation of uninvolved tissues is critical for cosmesis and function. It also works well for irregularly shaped tumors to ensure clear margins. It provides greater than 95% cure rates for BCC and greater than 92% cure rates for SCC. Defects can be closed primarily, by flap closure, by skin graft, or by secondary intervention depending on the size and location.[9]

Nonsurgical destructive techniques include cryosurgery and electrodessication. These techniques should be used judiciously for smaller superficial lesions, because they do not provide surgical specimens for histopathologic analysis. In addition, these are best used in noncritical locations where cosmesis is not a concern, because by design, they produce wounds that heal by secondary intention. The local failure rate is high.

SCC may also be treated using medical therapy. Radiation has been used as a primary modality for cutaneous SCC, with success rates of up to 90%. The side effects of dermatitis and fibrosis are not insignificant, however, and this modality is therefore best reserved for patients unable or unwilling to undergo surgery. The debilitated patient with comorbid medical disease, for example, may pose a sufficient enough anesthesia risk for surgical intervention that the risks of radiation therapy are less morbid. Radiation therapy has also been used successfully as adjuvant therapy for large, high-stage, and/or recurrent tumors.

Photodynamic therapy (PDT) has been approved in the United States for the treatment of actinic keratoses. Off-label use extends to treatment for BCC. This process involves the application of porphyrins such as 5-aminolevulinic acid to a neoplastic lesion and then photoexciting the molecules with specific wavelengths of light. The energy produced is transferred to neighboring oxygen molecules that form singlet oxygen free radicals, which in turn destroy adjacent tissue.

Topical 5-fluorouracil (5-FU), an antimetabolite, is used frequently to treat premalignant lesions such as actinic keratoses. Although it is a good choice in that regard, it is not recommended as primary treatment of cutaneous SCC. Topical imiquimod may also be used for multiple AK, as can laser and chemical skin resurfacing.

BASAL CELL CANCER
Basal Cell Cancer Epidemiology

BCC, like SCC, is a disease of sun exposure. It is the most common type of skin cancer in the United States. It is far more common than SCC and accounts for approximately 75% of all nonmelanoma skin cancers. Tumors affect men with a 3:2 predilection. Short-wave UVB radiation is the most likely culprit in pathogenesis. Like SCC, it tends to occur mostly on the head, neck, and other sun-exposed areas. It is one of the most common cancers in the United States, developing primarily in fair-skinned and light-eyed individuals with a history of intense sun exposure. Unlike SCC, it is slow growing and rarely metastasizes. It does, however, cause extensive morbidity through local tissue destruction in critical areas, particularly the face. Other risk factors for the development of BCC include a history of x-ray radiation, arsenic exposure, a prior history of nonmelanoma skin cancer, xeroderma pigmentosum, and nevoid BCC syndrome. Nevoid BCC syndrome or Gorlin-Goltz syndrome is a rare autosomal dominant disorder causing a characteristic facies, skeletal anomalies, symptomatic jaw cysts, and numerous BCC from birth or early childhood.

Diagnosis

BCC is typically a disease of elderly light-skinned individuals, given the link with chronic sun exposure. Lesions are slow growing, so they often come to attention only after significant disfigurement or local trauma and bleeding are encountered. There are several subtypes of BCC, each of varying degrees of aggression.

- Nodular
- Pigmented
- Cystic
- Superficial
- Micronodular
- Morpheaform (infiltrating)

Nodular BCC is the most common subtype of BCC. It forms a waxy or pearly appearing papule with raised, well-demarcated borders. One can often see telangiectasias over the translucent surface or central ulceration and crusting that bleeds with minor trauma.

Pigmented BCC can be mistaken for melanoma because of the increased content of brown or black pigment (in addition to the features of nodular BCC). These BCC occur more frequently in darker-skinned people.

Cystic BCC is marked by bluish or gray cystic nodules that may be misidentified as benign cysts.

Superficial BCC takes on a scaly patch-like or papule form that varies in color from pink to red or brown. Erosion is less common, and these lesions rarely become invasive. Psoriasis and eczema can be mistaken diagnoses for these lesions, which occur more commonly on the trunk.

Micronodular BCC is an aggressive variant of BCC, which appears to have well-defined border and is less prone to ulceration.

Morpheaform and infiltrating BCC are also aggressive BCC variants. Unlike other subtypes, they usually have ill-defined borders that extend beyond clinically visible margins. They have an almost scar-like appearance in a plaque or papule formation that can in fact be mistaken for scar tissue. Ulceration, bleeding, and crusting are uncommon. They require wider margins to ensure complete resection.[5]

Histopathology

BCCs originate from the pluripotential epithelial cells of the epidermis and hair follicles. UVB damage to the tumor suppressor genes of these cells leads to carcinogenesis through the hedgehog signaling pathway. BCC can also be seen in genetic syndromes, again as a result of defects in tumor suppressor gene function. BCCs are typically slow-growing tumors that take months to years to reach a size sufficient for a patient to seek care. On microscopy, cells stain basophilic, have a prominent nucleus, and form orderly linear patterns or "palisades" around nests of dermal tumor cells. The "rodent ulcer" was so named by Arthur Jacob in 1827 to describe the central necrosis that eventually occurs in longstanding lesions. He also noted that lesions recurred frequently despite apparent clinical excision, attesting to the insidious tissue destruction that occurs by direct tumor extension.

Treatment

Surgical treatment

Surgical treatment for BCC as for SCC employs Mohs microsurgery technique as well as direct surgical excision. Excision margins are recommended to be from 2 to 10 mm, less than the 4 to 15 mm recommended for SCC. Analysis of studies performed to investigate the correlation between margin status and recurrence reveal that, indeed, recurrence is directly related to adequacy of resection. In one study, negative margins of 0.5 mm or more result in a 1.2% recurrence rate, whereas positive margins result in up to 33% recurrence rates over a 5-year interval. Based on retrospective studies of recurrence rates, visual margins of 2 mm for subcentimeter lesions and 4 mm for greater than 1 cm lesions have been recommended.[10,11]

Nonsurgical treatment

Cryosurgery and electrodessication, as with SCC, are useful tools in the nonsurgical management of BCC. Cure rates of up to 90% have been cited with cryosurgery, though this treatment modality may leave unpredictable scars after the necrosis and swelling resolves. It also has the disadvantage of not providing a specimen for histopathologic analysis of margins. Lesions of less than 6 to 10 mm on the head and neck or 20 mm on the trunk and extremities are best suited for destructive techniques or direct surgical excision. Mohs surgery and radiation are appropriate options for larger lesions where tissue preservation is critical.

Topical treatment for BCC is similar to that of SCC. 5-FU and imiquimod have been used successfully to treat small, superficial BCC. 5-FU is a good choice for patients with basal cell nevus syndrome who may have subclinical BCC at any given time. PDT has been used in off-label purposes to treat BCC. Intralesional interferon-alpha 2b has not gained mainstream favor because of the cost and inconvenience associated with therapy.

MELANOMA

Epidemiology

Melanoma comprises only 4% to 5% of all skin cancers, but it is responsible for the majority of deaths from skin cancer. There were 62,480 new diagnoses of cutaneous melanoma in 2008, with a slightly greater distribution in men than that in women. Melanoma mortality numbered 8420, again with a higher distribution in men. Unlike with nonmelanoma skin cancers, the occurrence of melanoma correlates more with the intensity of prior sun exposure than cumulative exposure. A history of five or more sunburns in early life has been associated with a doubled risk of developing malignant melanoma later in life. Other risk factors include fair skin and light eyes, dysplastic nevi, multiple (>50) nevi, prior history of melanoma, family history of melanoma, weakened immune system (transplant patient), and xeroderma pigmentosum. Tumors tend to appear more often on lower extremities in women and on the head, neck, and trunk in men. Melanomas, unlike NMSC, do not necessarily restrict themselves to appearing in sun-exposed areas and may arise in unusual locations such as in the subungual and perianal regions.[12]

Precursor Lesions

The development of melanoma has been associated with congenital nevi, Spitz nevi, and dysplastic nevi. Small congenital nevi (<1.5 cm) are at low risk for malignant transformation, because they often do not contain melanocytes in the deeper dermis. Prophylactic removal is not recommended. Giant congenital nevi (>20 cm), although rare, do carry a 5% to 8% risk of developing malignant melanoma within the nevi.

Half of these occur in early childhood, so if possible, excision has been recommended for thick lesions. Intermediate lesions may be followed clinically with biopsies performed on deeper appearing or otherwise suspicious areas.

Spitz nevi typically occur in children and are also known as juvenile melanoma, spindle cell melanoma, and epithelioid melanoma. These lesions appear pink or brown because of their high vascularity. They are benign, but they grow rapidly and may be difficult to differentiate from malignant melanoma on histologic analysis. Local excision with margins is recommended, as if one were treating melanoma if the diagnosis is in question.[13]

Dysplastic nevi are large pigmented lesions of variable color and indistinct border. Most will not develop into melanomas, but a family history of melanoma or dysplastic nevus syndrome (>100 nevi) confers an increased risk. These patients require close follow-up with a physician for routine 3- to 6-month surveillance for both occurrence of new lesions and transformation of existing lesions. Photographs can be a good way to evaluate and record change.

Familial melanoma describes a subgroup of patients (5%–10%) who have a prior family history of melanoma. They tend to be affected at an earlier age than patients who develop sporadic melanoma, and they tend to have both multiple primaries as well as dysplastic nevi.[14,15]

Histopathology

Melanocytes derive from neural crest tissue, which migrates to the dermal-epidermal junction. Development of melanoma is associated with exposure to UV radiation or malignant transformation of precursor lesions. Five histologic subtypes of melanoma exist:

- Superficial spreading melanoma (SSM)
- Nodular melanoma (NM)
- Lentigo maligna melanoma (LMM)
- Acral lentiginous melanoma (ALM)
- Desmoplastic melanoma (DM)

Classification is based on growth pattern and location. NM differs from the other subtypes in that the vertical growth phase occurs early, whereas the others expand radially first. This vertical component of growth is the most important histopathologic factor determining prognosis.

SSM is the most common subtype of melanoma, accounting for 70% of lesions. LMM tends to occur in an older patient population and grows slowly and superficially. NM has the worst prognosis because of the prominence of the vertical growth phase; this tends to be thicker at diagnosis. ALM is located in the subungual regions and in the glabrous skin of the palms and soles, typically in patients of African American descent. It is an easy to miss diagnosis, leading to a poor prognosis based on delay in treatment. DM is a rare but aggressive subtype of melanoma notable for its propensity toward perineural invasion and recurrence. DMs occur mostly on the head and neck of elderly men in their sixth and seventh decades of life and are often deep at the time of diagnosis given the difficulty of clinical diagnosis with these atypical and often unpigmented lesions.

Diagnosis

The ABCD rule evaluates lesions suspicious for melanoma. A refers to Asymmetry, B to border irregularity, C to color (uneven), and D to diameter greater than 6 mm. Pain, itching, bleeding, swelling, and appearance of new nodules can also be associated with malignant melanoma.

Melanoma is staged according to the American Joint Committee on Cancer TNM (Tumor, Node, Metastases) classification, which takes into account several features: the extent of primary tumor as determined by tumor depth, presence of ulceration, lymph node status, and presence or absence of metastasis. Tumor depth is evaluated by Breslow depth, a measurement of tumor thickness from top to base in millimeters and by Clark's level (**Table 1**), which defines the level of invasion into the distinct layers of dermis and subcutaneous fat. Using Breslow depth, T1 lesions measure less than or equal to 1.0 mm; T2 lesions, from 1.01 to 2.0 mm; T3 lesions, from 2.01 to 4.0 mm; and lesions greater than 4.0 mm in depth are considered T4 lesions.

Tumor ulceration refers to the presence or absence of intact epidermis overlying the primary lesion bases on microscopic examination. Ulceration indicates a more aggressive tumor, putting survival rates into a category similar to that of a patient with a nonulcerated tumor of the next T category. Lymph node status has been refined into macroscopic and microscopic categories by the advent of sentinel lymph node biopsy and immunohistochemical staining for melanocytes. A high mitotic index is also indicative of more aggressive tumors.

The most important factor in staging melanoma is tumor depth. It is imperative that lesions undergo excisional or full-thickness biopsy with narrow 1- to 2-mm margins encompassing the lesion and extending into subcutaneous fat to preserve this critical staging information. The tissue should be handled atraumatically, with avoidance of electrocautery to allow most accurate histologic analysis. The resulting wound should be closed in an orientation that will minimize tissue loss and facilitate closure in the event of reexcision. A lesion undergoing biopsy for suspicion of melanoma should never be shave-biopsied or manipulated in a way that would compromise the evaluation of depth.[16]

Patients presenting with a new diagnosis of melanoma should undergo a thorough history and physical examination, including full skin examination. The components of history include documentation of patient's phenotype, history of blistering sunburns, occupation-/travel-related sun exposure, and family history of melanoma. Physical examination should include head to toe skin examination, including perianal skin. Nodal basins should be palpated for evidence of metastases as well as examining surrounding tissues for evidence of in-transit metastases.

Treatment

Surgical treatment

The mainstay of treatment for malignant melanoma is wide surgical excision with appropriate margins. For in situ lesions, a margin of 0.5 cm is considered adequate. Lesions of

Table 1	
Clark's level tumor invasiveness measurement	
Clark's Level	**Location of Tumor**
I	Epidermis only (in situ)
II	Into papillary dermis
III	To base of papillary dermis
IV	Into reticular dermis
V	Into subcutaneous tissue

less than 1 mm Breslow depth require 1-cm margins. Lesions from 1 to 2 mm can be resected with 1-cm margins if necessary to allow for primary closure or to avoid critical structures; 2 cm is recommended. Lesions of greater than 2 mm Breslow depth require 2-cm margins; larger margins have not been shown to give a significant advantage in retrospective reviews. It is important to remember that margin excisions should be measured from the ends of the biopsy scar; oftentimes, biopsy removes the clinically apparent tumor. It is imperative, therefore, that initial biopsy includes specimen orientation and that the size of that incision is conservative. Subungual melanomas can be treated by distal phalanx amputation, which gives a 1-cm margin of normal tissue.

Sentinel lymph node biopsy has made rapid advances in the detection of metastatic melanoma and minimized the morbidity associated with unnecessary lymph node dissection. It is now a recommended staging procedure for lesions greater than 1 mm in thickness or shallower lesions that have poor prognostic characteristics such as ulceration.[12]

Nonsurgical treatment

Interferon alpha-2b has shown some success in treating patients with nodal or in-transit metastasis or node-negative thick melanoma (>4 mm). It is of indeterminate value for intermediate lesions (2–4 mm). Much research is ongoing in the field of immunotherapy to develop melanoma vaccines, but as of now, these are costly, difficult to translate to mainstream therapy, and of limited access.

SUMMARY

Cutaneous malignancies are extremely common clinical entities that will be encountered by the general surgeon in practice today. The general surgeon should understand the role sun exposure plays in the development of basal cell, squamous cell, and melanoma skin cancers to accurately diagnose and counsel affected and at-risk patients. Other risk factors for carcinogenesis, such as immunosuppression and chronic wounds, also fall under the domain of general surgical care; vigilant surveillance must be maintained for abnormal lesions when caring for these patients. Attention must be given to surgical principles of appropriate resection margins and specimen orientation when operating on these patients. In summary, general surgeons serve an important role both in the primary care of patients with common cutaneous malignancies as well as in facilitating the referral system between primary care physician, plastic surgeon, dermatologist, and oncologist.

REFERENCES

1. Available at: http://seer.cancer.gov/cgi-bin/csr/1975_2005/search.pl#results. Accessed August 19, 2008.
2. Vincent T DeVita, Samuel Hellman, Steven A. Rosenberg. Cancer: principles & practice of oncology, 7th edition. Baltimore, MD: Lippincott Williams & Wilkins, 2005.
3. Colver G, Bill Bowers B. Skin cancer: a practical guide to surgical management. Informa Health Care; 2002.
4. Available at: http://www.cancer.gov/cancertopics/types/skin. Accessed August 19, 2008.
5. Carucci JA, Leffell DJ. Basal cell carcinoma. Fitzpatrick's dermatology in general medicine. 6th edition. New York: McGraw-Hill; 2003. p. 737–47, 747–54.
6. Grossman D, Leffell DJ. Squamous cell carcinoma. Fitzpatrick's dermatology in general medicine. 6th edition. New York: McGraw-Hill; 2003. p. 747–54.

7. Tan PY, Ek E, Su S, et al. Incomplete excision of squamous cell carcinoma of the skin: a prospective observational study. Plast Reconstr Surg 2007;120(4):910–6.
8. Mohs FE. Chemosurgery for skin cancer: fixed and fresh tissue techniques. Arch Dermatol 1976;112(2):211–5.
9. Mohs FE. Chemosurgery. Clin Plast Surg 1980;7(3):349–60.
10. Thomas DJ, King AR, Peat BG. Excision margins for nonmelanotic skin cancer. Plast Reconstr Surg 2003;112(1):57–63.
11. Ross MI. New American Joint Commission on cancer staging system for melanoma: prognostic impact and future directions. Surg Oncol Clin N Am 2006; 15(2):341–52.
12. Urist MM, Soong S. Melanoma and cutaneous malignancies. In: Townsend CM, Beauchamp RD, Evers BM, editors. Townsend: sabiston textbook of surgery. 18th edition. Philadelphia: Saunders; 2007.
13. Habif TP. Premalignant and malignant nonmelanoma skin tumors. In: Clinical dermatology. 4th edition. Edinburgh: Mosby, Inc; 2004.
14. Habif TP. Nevi and malignant melanoma. In: Clinical dermatology. 4th edition. Edinburgh: Mosby, Inc; 2004.
15. Smoller BR. Squamous cell carcinoma: from precursor lesions to high-risk variants. Mod Pathol 2006;19:S88–92.
16. Final version of the American Joint Committee on cancer staging system for cutaneous melanoma. J Clin Oncol 2001;19:3635–48. Lippincott Williams & Wilkins.

Current Concepts in Cutaneous Melanoma: Malignant Melanoma

Andrew R. Doben, MD[a],*, Dougald C. MacGillivray, MD, FACS[b]

KEYWORDS

- Melanoma • Neoplasm staging • Sentinel node biopsy
- Pigmented skin lesions • Nodal evaluation

INCIDENCE

Melanoma of the skin is one of the most clinically important skin and soft tissue lesions encountered by the practicing general surgeon. If properly diagnosed and treated in its early stages, its prognosis and outcome are uniformly favorable.[1] Data from the National Cancer Institute (NCI) estimates that 62,480 new cases of melanoma of the skin are diagnosed in the United States each year (34,950 men and 27,530 women). Approximately 8420 of these patients will die from their disease.[1]

The disease has a predilection toward individuals aged 30 to 70 years, which is likely related to lifetime sun exposure; however, all ages are affected to some degree, confirming the multifactorial nature of the malignancy. Between 1970 and 1990 the incidence of melanoma increased steadily, but now seems to be slowing due to general public awareness and consequent reduced exposure to UV light.[2] (p3) According to national statistics from 2001 to 2005, the median age at diagnosis for melanoma of the skin was 59 years (**Table 1**).[1]

Based on the National Surveillance, Epidemiology, and End Results (SEER) database, the age-adjusted incidence rate was 19.4 per 100,000 men and women per year.[1] A slightly higher incidence seems to occur in individuals with lighter skin, again confirming that UV damage and sun exposure are relative risk factors (**Table 2**).

From 2001 to 2005, the median age at death from melanoma of the skin was 68 years.[1] There is a slight trend toward increasing mortality in patients with melanoma, and older age is a predictor of poorer survival. These data have been reviewed in numerous trials and were reported in the 2003 review of cutaneous melanoma in The Surgical Clinics of North America.[2] In 2004, Chao and colleagues published a retrospective study confirming that age is an independent prognostic indicator of poor overall survival. Chao and colleagues were also were able to extract data from

[a] Department of Surgery, Maine Medical Center, Division of Surgical Oncology, 22 Bramhall Street, Portland, ME 04102, USA
[b] The Maine Surgical Care Group, 887 Congress Street, Portland, ME 04102, USA
* Corresponding author.
E-mail address: adoben@gmail.com (A.R. Doben).

Surg Clin N Am 89 (2009) 713–725
doi:10.1016/j.suc.2009.03.003
0039-6109/09/$ – see front matter © 2009 Elsevier Inc. All rights reserved.

surgical.theclinics.com

Table 1
Age distribution of new cases of melanoma

Age Distribution (y)	Percentage of Annual Cases (%)
<20	0.9
20–34	8.1
35–44	12.9
45–54	18.9
55–64	19.5
65–74	17.8
75–84	16.4
85+	5.5

Data from National Cancer Institute. Surveillance, epidemiology, and end results (SEER), 17 September 2008. National Institutes of Health SEER, US National Institutes of Health. Available at: http://seer.cancer.gov/statfacts/html/melan.html.

the Sunbelt Melanoma trial.[3] The results of the analysis revealed that as age increases more adverse features of melanoma are also present, including Breslow thickness, ulceration, and proportion of male patients.[4] All of these factors are known to contribute to increased mortality (**Table 3**).

One of the most important aspects of long-term survival and prognosis is stage at diagnosis, which confirms that early detection and proper therapy play an important role in the treatment of melanoma. Five-year survival is greatly affected by the distribution of the disease at the time of diagnosis (**Table 4**). Currently, 93% of all melanomas are diagnosed at early stage of disease, which confers much greater survival.

EVALUATION

The initial evaluation of all patients who present with pigmented skin lesions should be methodical. The importance of a detailed history and physical examination cannot be emphasized enough, even in a busy practice environment. Special attention should be given to a personal history of early and harsh sun exposure. Accounts of blistering sunburns either as a small child or teenager should raise suspicion, as should multiple lesions excised by a dermatologist or other medical specialist for what patients may describe as abnormal but not malignant lesions, as well as reports of changing skin lesions.

Table 2
Incidence of melanoma by race

Race/Ethnicity	Males per 100,000	Females per 100,000
All races	24.6	15.6
White	28.5	18.5
Black	1.1	0.9
Asian/Pacific Islander	1.6	1.3
American Indian/Alaska Native	3.9	2.6
Hispanic	4.8	4.9

Data from National Cancer Institute. Surveillance, epidemiology, and end results (SEER), 17 September 2008. National Institutes of Health SEER, US National Institutes of Health. Available at: http://seer.cancer.gov/statfacts/html/melan.html.

Table 3 Age-based mortality	
Age Distribution (y)	Death Rate (%)
<20	0.1
20–34	2.9
35–44	7.2
45–54	15.0
55–64	18.8
65–74	21.3
75–84	23.6
85+	11.0[11]

Data from National Cancer Institute. Surveillance, epidemiology, and end results (SEER), 17 September 2008. National Institutes of Health SEER, US National Institutes of Health, Available at: http://seer.cancer.gov/statfacts/html/melan.html.

A family history of skin malignancies or melanoma is of utmost importance. Age at diagnosis in the family member and the location of the lesion (truncal vs extremity) and their current health status should be noted at the initial screening.

Directed questions and physical examination for recognizing the hallmarks of melanoma, or what has been previously described as the ABCDEs of melanoma, should follow.

A. Asymmetry—different halves of the skin lesion do not look the same
B. Borders—irregular, shaggy, or badly formed
C. Color—not the same throughout the lesion
D. Diameter—larger than 6 mm
E. Evolving—change in the size, shape, shades of color, symptoms (itching, tenderness), or surface (especially bleeding)[5,c]

In addition, the physical examination should involve a thorough evaluation of all potential draining lymph node basins based on lesion location. Clinically palpable lymph nodes indicate an important branch point in a decision tree algorithm.

DIAGNOSIS

Appropriate diagnosis of all suspicious skin lesions requires histologic tissue diagnosis on permanent section. In conjunction with other immunohistologic chemical staining, histologic tissue diagnosis is the gold standard for diagnosis. A shave biopsy

Table 4 Dissemination of disease at presentation and 5-year survival		
Disease Pattern	Distribution at Diagnosis (%)	5-Year Survival Rate (%)
Localized	81	98.7
Regional spread	12	65.1
Distant metastasis	4	15.5
Unknown stage	4	77.4

---

[c] Elevation is a newer method of evaluation, popularized since the JAMA article[5] in 2004.

of the lesion is inappropriate to properly microstage melanoma. Any lesion that is suspicious for a cutaneous malignancy should undergo a full-thickness biopsy.

Incisional Versus Excisional Biopsy

For small pigmented lesions that are not highly suspicious for melanoma, the initial full-thickness biopsy may be diagnostic and therapeutic. Using Langer lines (**Fig. 1**), a full-thickness excision (down to the layer of the muscular fascia) with normal skin margins of 1 to 4 mm is an appropriate first step. The specimen should be marked for orientation.[6] If the lesion is not amenable to an excisional biopsy, a full-thickness

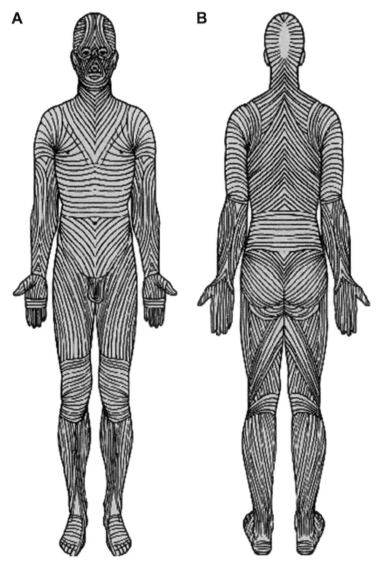

Fig. 1. (*A, B*) Langer lines. (*From* Dorland's illustrated medical dictionary. 31st edition. Philadelphia: Saunders Elsevier; 2007. p. 1069.)

punch or incisional biopsy is appropriate. Neither incisional nor punch biopsy increases the risk of recurrence or metastasis. Should the biopsy confirm a melanoma, data obtained from the pathology report are important determinants of treatment planning and final therapy.

Pathologic Evaluation

Histologic evaluation of the surgical specimen is presented in the final pathology report. All pigmented lesions should be reported in a similar fashion. The following list of pathologic features is recommended as standard for final pathology reports by the National Comprehensive Cancer Network (NCCN) (**Fig. 2**):

1. Growth pattern – this is typically defined as radial versus vertical. A vertical growth pattern confers more malignant potential
2. Histologic subtype – four main subtypes have been reported
   a. Lentigo maligna—only 5% of cases
   b. Superficial spreading—approximately 70% of cases
   c. Acral lentiginous—approximately 10% of cases
   d. Nodular melanoma—approximately 15% to 30% of cases
   e. Desmoplastic melanoma—a rare subtype
3. Clark level of invasion
   a. Level 1
   b. Level 2
   c. Level 3
   d. Level 4
   e. Level 5
4. Breslow thickness in millimeters (depth of invasion)
5. Ulceration
6. Mitotic index
7. Angiolymphatic invasion
8. Tumor infiltrating lymphocyte activity (TIL)
9. Neurotropism

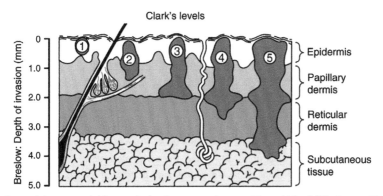

Fig. 2. Dermal layers and histopathologic nomenclature. (*From* Urist MM, Soong SJ. Melanoma and cutaneous malignancies. In: Townsend Jr. CM, Beauchamp RD, Evers M, et al., editors. Sabiston textbook of surgery: the biological basis of modern surgical practice, vol. 1. 18th edition. Philadelphia: Saunders; 2008. p. 771; with permission.)

Once the final tissue diagnosis has confirmed melanoma, additional staging and surgical evaluation should continue.

STAGING

The American Joint Committee on Cancer (AJCC) TNM Clinical Classification of Melanoma, 6th edition (2002), is well established.[7] **Tables 5–7** outline the AJCC staging components based on clinical and pathologic evaluation. This TNM model is then classified into further stages in **Table 8**.

The T stage of the classification is based primarily on tumor depth in conjunction with adverse features, specifically ulceration (see **Table 5**).

The N section of staging is determined by involvement of either regional or distant lymph nodes. The N staging is determined from the pathologic specimen (ie, sentinel node, fine-needle aspiration [FNA], or regional nodal resection) or clinically detectable disease (ie, palpable nodes or radiographically positive nodes) (see **Table 6**).

The M portion of the staging criteria is usually based on clinical or radiographic findings. If distant lesions are present either clinically or radiographically and are suspicious for metastatic disease, pathologic tissue evaluation should be obtained whenever possible.[7] However, tissue biopsy is not an absolute requirement for M staging (see **Table 7**).

The TNM staging criteria are based on a combination of pathologic and clinical staging. The final stage is based on the summative TNM staging from the AJCC sixth edition (2002) descriptions. Certain histologic findings upstage lesions because these characteristics are poor prognostic indicators. Ulceration has historically been one such entity. However. recent data[8] suggest that ulceration may be a surrogate for melanoma proliferative activity and that the mitotic index may be a more important indicator of tumor virulence. At the time of publication of this article, the mitotic index

Table 5 AJCC T staging criteria	
Tumor Stage	**Pathologic Features**
TX	Primary tumor cannot be assessed (ie, shave biopsy)
T0	No evidence of primary tumor
Tis	Melanoma in situ
T1	Melanoma ≤1.0 mm thick with or without ulceration
T1a	Melanoma ≤1.0 mm thick and Clark level II or III, no ulceration
T1b	Melanoma ≤1.0 mm thick and Clark level IV or V or with ulceration
T2	Melanoma 1.01–2.0 mm thick with or without ulceration
T2a	Melanoma 1.01–2.0 mm thick with no ulceration
T2b	Melanoma 1.01–2.0 mm thick with ulceration
T3	Melanoma 2.01–4.0 mm thick with or without ulceration
T3a	Melanoma 2.01–4.0 mm thick with no ulceration
T3b	Melanoma 2.01–4.0 mm thick with ulceration
T4	Melanoma >4.0 mm thick with or without ulceration
T4a	Melanoma >4.0 mm thick with no ulceration
T4b	Melanoma >4.0 mm thick with ulceration

Data from The American Joint Committee on Cancer (AJCC). TNM clinical classification of melanoma. 6th edition. AJCC; 2002.

Table 6	
AJCC N staging criteria	
Regional Lymph Nodes	**Nodal Evaluation**
NX	Regional lymph nodes cannot be assessed
N0	No regional lymph node metastasis
N1	Metastasis in 1 lymph node
N1a	Clinically occult (microscopic) metastasis
N1b	Clinically apparent (macroscopic) metastasis
N2	Metastasis in 2 or 3 regional nodes or intralymphatic regional metastasis without nodal metastases
N2a	Clinically occult (microscopic) metastasis
N2b	Clinically apparent (macroscopic) metastasis
N2c	Satellite or in-transit metastasis without nodal metastasis
N3	Metastasis in 4 or more regional nodes, matted metastatic nodes, in-transit metastasis, or satellites with metastasis in regional node(s)

Data from The American Joint Committee on Cancer (AJCC). TNM clinical classification of melanoma. 6th edition. AJCC; 2002.

was not featured as a component of the TNM classification. This is likely to change in the upcoming revisions of the TNM classification from the AJCC.

Pathologic staging is important to the clinician and the patient. Most survival data are reported by pathologic stage, and appropriately staging the patient classifies their tumor and their treatment by evidence-based practice. Staging also helps to determine those patients who will be candidates for clinical trials.

TREATMENT

Once a final tissue diagnosis has been confirmed, the most important determinant in further management is based on pathologic microstaging. The mainstay of treatment of melanoma is surgical, with 2 specific goals:

1. Excision of the primary lesion with appropriate margins
2. Evaluation of the nodal basin for staging and disease clearance

Table 7	
AJCC M staging criteria	
Distant Metastasis	**Staging Findings**
MX	Distant metastasis cannot be assessed
M0	No distant metastasis
M1	Distant metastasis
M1a	Metastasis to skin, subcutaneous tissue, or distant lymph nodes
M1b	Metastasis to lung
M1c	Metastasis to all other visceral sites or distant metastasis at any site associated with elevated serum lactate dehydrogenase

From The American Joint Committee on Cancer (AJCC) TNM clinical classification of melanoma. 6th edition. AJCC; 2002.

Table 8
AJCC melanoma staging

Pathologic Stage	Tumor	Node	Metastasis
0	Tis	N0	M0
IA	T1a	N0	M0
IB	T1b	N0	M0
	T2a	N0	M0
IIA	T2b	N0	M0
	T3a	N0	M0
IIB	T3b	N0	M0
	T4a	N0	M0
IIC	T4b	N0	M0
IIIA	T1–4a	N1a	M0
	T1–4a	N2a	M0
IIIB	T1–4b	N1a	M0
	T1–4b	N2a	M0
	T1–4a	N1b	M0
	T1–4a	N2b	M0
	T1–4a/b	N2c	M0
IIIC	T1–4b	N1b	M0
	T1–4b	N2b	M0
	Any T	N3	M0
IV	Any T	Any N	M1

From The American Joint Committee on Cancer (AJCC) TNM clinical classification of melanoma. 6th edition. AJCC; 2002.

There have been numerous prospective randomized trials that support the recommendations for margins of the primary lesion and the evaluation of the nodal basin as described earlier. The current NCCN guidelines, available at http://www.nccn.org, are based on these trials.

In Situ Melanoma (Stage 0)

In situ melanoma should be excised using a 0.5-cm margin from all edges of either the lesion or the prior surgical site. With in situ disease (Stage 0), excision is the sole treatment.

Lesions <1.0 mm Breslow Tumor Thickness (Stage IA)

For lesions that are less than 1.0 mm by Breslow tumor thickness and a Clark level II or III, wide local excision with a 1.0-cm margin is the sole treatment.

Lesions <1.0 mm Breslow Tumor Thickness with Adverse Features (Stage IB and IIA)

Thin lesions, <1.0 mm in depth of Breslow tumor thickness, with adverse features or Clark level thickness IV or V, have a low, but real risk for occult nodal metastasis (ie, Stage IB and Stage IIA lesions). These tumors should be resected with wide local excision of 1.0 cm from all margins and sentinel lymph node (SLN) evaluation should be considered.[9]

Lesions Between 1.01 mm and 2.0 mm Breslow Tumor Thickness (Stage IB and IIA)

Lesions between 1.01 mm and 2.0 mm of Breslow tumor thickness require wide local excision with margins of 1.0 to 2.0 cm from all tumor edges based on the ability to achieve primary closure. Patients with these lesions without clinical evidence of regional nodal disease should undergo sentinel lymph node evaluation.

Lesions >2.01 mm Breslow Tumor Thickness (Stage IIA and Higher)

Initial surgical specimens with Breslow tumor thickness of 2.01 mm or deeper should undergo wide local excision with 2.0 cm radial margins from all tumor or prior surgical excision margins. Patients with these lesions without clinical evidence of regional nodal disease or metastatic disease from staging studies should undergo sentinel lymph node evaluation.

Management of Lymph Nodes

The use of sentinel lymph node[d] biopsy in melanoma is accepted as an appropriate method of accurately staging individuals who may have occult nodal metastasis. To date no randomized prospective studies have demonstrated overall survival benefit comparing patients who have had a sentinel node biopsy versus those who have had nodal observation. However, the Multicenter Selective Lymphadenectomy Trial (MSLT) I demonstrated that patients who had a positive sentinel lymph node and who underwent immediate lymphadenectomy had a significant 5-year survival advantage over those patients who were observed and had a lymphadenectomy only after developing clinically evident lymphadenopathy.[10] MSLT II, in which individuals with a positive SLN biopsy are randomized to completion lymphadenectomy versus observation, is underway. This study will hopefully clearly delineate if there is an overall survival benefit to immediate therapeutic lymphadenectomy following a positive sentinel lymph node biopsy. With the current AJCC staging model, all individuals with a Stage Ib or higher melanoma without clinically positive lymph nodes should be offered a sentinel lymph node biopsy (**Fig. 3**).[11]

Clinically Detectable Lymph Nodes

Any patient with either a biopsy-proven melanoma or a pigmented lesion highly suspicious for malignant melanoma with clinically palpable lymph nodes should be considered to have regional disease. Biopsy-proven melanoma of any stage, with palpable lymph nodes, should raise the suspicion of the clinician to consider a detailed evaluation. Nodal evaluation by ultrasound with fine-needle aspiration should precede surgical intervention. If surgically resectable, wide local excision of the primary lesion and complete regional lymphadenectomy is indicated. Further staging with additional imaging for potential metastatic disease should be performed.

A complete lymph node dissection should include an anatomically complete dissection of the entire nodal basin involved. In the axilla this is usually a Level I and II axillary dissection. Although deep nodal dissections remain controversial, NCCN

---

[d] It has been well supported in the literature that sentinel lymph node (SLN) evaluation is equivalent in its ability to detect micrometastatic melanoma to elective lymph node dissection. The appropriate identification of the SLN by surgeons experienced in this technique is between 90 and 100%. Therefore it is possible to safely identify those individuals who may benefit from regional lymphadenectomy without subjecting all patients to this potentially morbid procedure. Numerous studies have verified that in those areas of the body in which the nodal basin is reasonably predictable, specifically the extremities, the accuracy of SLN biopsy is significantly higher. Although recent studies have not clearly shown inferiority, the accuracy of SLN biopsy can be suspect in locations in which the nodal basin is less predictable.

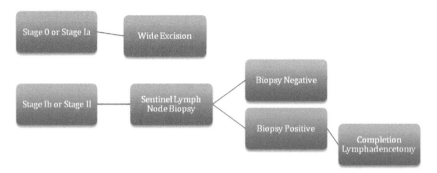

Fig. 3. Early stage disease surgical algorithm. (*Data from* National Comprehensive Cancer Network. Cutaneous melanoma guidelines, one January 2004. Available at: www.nccn. org.)

recommendations (based on category 2 evidence), suggest there may be benefit from a deep nodal dissection in some patients. Some sources recommend deep nodal dissection of the groin in patients with at least one of the following:

1. ≥3 superficial positive nodes (based on category 2B evidence)
2. Pelvic CT is positive for iliac and obturator lymphadenopathy (category 2A evidence)
3. Cloquet[e] node is positive (category 2b evidence)[9]

Therapeutic Options Based on Staging

Adjuvant therapy
Currently interferon-α2B is the only adjuvant therapy regimen for malignant melanoma approved by the Food and Drug Administration. Over the past 2 decades, numerous studies have evaluated the clinical efficacy of interferon therapy as adjuvant treatment of stage IIB and III melanoma after primary resection and nodal evaluation. Numerous evaluations with different dose regimens and timing have all concluded that although there is an extension of relapse-free state, overall survival to 12.6 years is equivalent.[12] A recent metaanalysis of 13 clinical trials by Wheatley and colleagues suggests that the use of interferon-α2B as adjuvant therapy may confer a significant relapse advantage and a small overall survival benefit (∼3%) compared with those who did not receive adjuvant therapy.[13]

The conclusion of most consensus groups remains that the use of interferon as an adjuvant therapy in the setting of Stage II or III cutaneous melanoma is undefined, and that use of such a regimen should be made on an individual patient basis.

Radiation therapy in Stage III and higher melanoma
For Stage IIIC disease, several retrospective studies have attempted to evaluate the use of radiotherapy on the nodal basin; however, the survival advantage (category 2B data) has not been shown in any prospective randomized data.[9] This is especially unclear for patients who have had a complete R0 resection of the primary lesion and the nodal basin.

---

[e] The first node under the inguinal ligament.

Stage IV and metastatic melanoma

Recommendations for treatment of Stage IV disease are based on initial staging and determination of the resectability of disease. If at the time of presentation it is established that the patient can undergo primary resection of the initial lesion in conjunction with the solitary distant disease, this should be attempted. Following surgery the patient should be offered adjuvant therapy with interferon-α2B or a clinical trial.[9]

Those patients who are not candidates for resection due to either widespread metastatic disease or incomplete resection should be treated with an advanced chemotherapy regimen or referred for clinical trial (**Fig. 4**).

Chemotherapy regimens

NCCN Practice Guidelines are available for worldwide review at www.nccn.org. These guidelines, reviewed annually, are based on current reviews of the literature by a panel of experts. According to category 2B recommendations from the literature, the following options are considered the standard of care for disseminated disease without brain metastasis (**Table 9**).

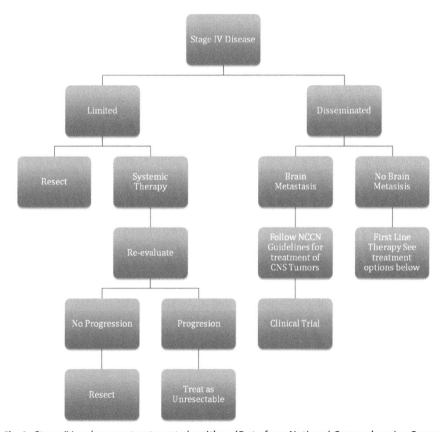

Fig. 4. Stage IV melanoma treatment algorithm. (*Data from* National Comprehensive Cancer Network. Cutaneous melanoma guidelines, 1 January 2004. Available at: www.nccn.org.)

Table 9 Chemotherapy regimen options^c	
Type of chemotherapy	Options
Single-agent chemotherapy	Dacarbazine, temozolomide, or paclitaxel, or high-dose interleukin-2
Combination chemotherapy	Paclitaxel with cisplatin or carboplatin
Combination chemotherapy or biochemotherapy	Dacarbazine or temozolomide-based including cisplatin and vinblastine, with or without interleukin-2, interferon-α

FURTHER READINGS

Balch CM, Soong S, Ross MI, et al. Long-term results of a multi-institutional randomized trial comparing prognostic factors and surgical results for intermediate thickness melanomas (1.0 to 4.0 mm). Intergroup Melanoma Surgical Trial. Ann Surg Oncol 2000;7(2):87–97.

Bickley LS, Hoekelman RA. Bates' guide to physical examination and history taking. 7th edition. Philadelphia: Lippincott Williams & Wilkins; 1999.

Newman Dorland WA. Dorland's illustrated medical dictionary. Philadelphia: Saunders Elsevier; 2007.

Doubrovsky A, de Wilt J, Scolyer R, et al. Sentinel node biopsy provides more accurate staging than elective lymph node dissection in patients. Ann Surg Oncol 2004; 11(9):829–36.

Essner R, Conforti A, Kelley MC, et al. Efficacy of lymphatic mapping, sentinel lymphadenectomy, and selective complete lymph node dissection as a therapeutic procedure for early-stage melanoma. Ann Surg Oncol 1999;6(5):442–9.

Gibbs JF, Huang PP, Zhang PJ, et al. Accuracy of pathologic techniques for the diagnosis of metastatic melanoma in sentinel lymph nodes. Ann Surg Oncol 1999;6(7): 699–704.

Kirkwood JM, Ibrahim JG, Sosman JA, et al. High-dose interferon alfa-2b significantly prolongs relapse-free and overall survival compared with the GM2-KLH/QS-21 vaccine in patients with resected stage IIB-III melanoma: results of Intergroup Trial E1694/S9512/C509801. J Clin Oncol 2001;19(9):2370–80.

Leong SPL. Malignant melanoma, part I. Surg Clin North Am 2003;83(1):1–29 97–107,109–56.

Muller M, Borgstein P, Pijpers R, et al. Reliability of the sentinel node procedure in melanoma patients: analysis of failures after long-term follow-up. Ann Surg Oncol 2000;7(6):461–8.

Torpy J. Melanoma. JAMA 2004;292(22):2800.

Urist MM, Soong S. Melanoma and Cutaneous Malignancies. In: Townsend CM Jr, Beauchamp RD, Evers M, et al, editors. Sabiston textbook of surgery: the biological basis of modern surgical practice, vol. 1. 18th edition. Philadelphia: Saunders; 2008. p. 767–80.

REFERENCES

1. National Cancer Institute. Surveillance, epidemiology, and end results (SEER), 17 September 2008. National Institutes of Health SEER, US National Institutes of Health. Available at: seer.cancer.gov. Accessed September 18, 2008.
2. Leong SPL. Malignant melanoma, part I. Surg Clin North Am 2003;83(1):3, 1–29.

3. McMasters K, Ross M, Reintgen D, et al. Final results of the Sunbelt Melanoma Trial. J Clin Oncol 2008;26(15 Suppl):9003 [meeting abstracts].
4. Chao C, Martin II MR, Ross MM, et al. Correlation between prognostic factors and increasing age in melanoma. Ann Surg Oncol 2004;11(3):259–64.
5. Abbasi NR. Early diagnosis of cutaneous melanoma: revisiting the ABCD criteria. JAMA 2004;292(22):2771–6.
6. Souba WW, et al. ACS surgery: principles & practice. 6th edition. New York: WebMD; 2007.
7. National Comprehensive Cancer Network. Cutaneous melanoma guidelines. Available at: www.nccn.org; 1 Jan 2004;. Accessed September 18, 2008.
8. Azzola MF, Shaw H, Thompson J, et al. Tumor mitotic rate is a more powerful prognostic indicator than ulceration in patients with primary cutaneous melanoma: an analysis of 3661 patients from a single center. Cancer 2003;97(6): 1488–98.
9. National Comprehensive Cancer Network. NCCN clinical practice guidelines in oncology: melanoma, clinical guidelines. Fort Washington (MD): National Comprehensive Cancer Network; 2009.
10. Morton DL, Thompson J, Cochran A, et al. Sentinel-node biopsy or nodal observation in melanoma. N Engl J Med 2006;355(13):1307–17.
11. Vaquerano J, Kraybill W, Driscoll D, et al. American Joint Committee on cancer clinical stage as a selection criterion for sentinel lymph node biopsy in thin melanoma. Ann Surg Oncol 2006;13(2):198–204.
12. Kirkwood JM, Ibrahim JG, Sondak VK, et al. Interferon alfa-2b adjuvant therapy of high-risk resected cutaneous melanoma: the Eastern Cooperative Oncology Group Trial EST 1684. J Clin Oncol 1996;14(1):7–17.
13. Wheatley K, et al. Interferon-alpha as adjuvant therapy for melanoma: an individual patient data meta-analysis of randomised trials. J Clin Oncol 2007;25(18 Suppl):8526 [meeting abstracts].

Unusual Skin Tumors: Merkel Cell Carcinoma, Eccrine Carcinoma, Glomus Tumors, and Dermatofibrosarcoma Protuberans

Jesse L. Kampshoff, MD[a], Thomas H. Cogbill, MD[b],*

KEYWORDS
- Merkel cell carcinoma • Eccrine carcinoma • Glomus tumors
- Dermatofibrosarcoma protuberans • Unusual skin tumors

MERKEL CELL CARCINOMA

In 1975, Friedrich Sigmond Merkel first described an epidermal, nondendritic, nonkeratinocyte cell that would later bear his name.[1] In 1972, Toker[2] described trabecular cell cancer of the skin; later evaluation with electron microscopy in 1978 suggested Merkel cell origin. The name Merkel cell carcinoma (MCC) was later coined by DeWolf-Peeters in 1980. The names trabecular cell carcinoma, primary small cell carcinoma of the skin, and anaplastic carcinoma of the skin all have been used to describe MCC.

Epidemiology

MCC is a rare, aggressive cutaneous malignancy that primarily affects older white persons. The average age at diagnosis is approximately 70 years. The incidence in white persons is 0.23 per 100,000, whereas in black persons it is 0.01 per 100,000. There are an estimated 470 new cases in the United States per year. Approximately 2000 cases have been reported in the literature. Incidence in men has been estimated at more than twice that in women.[1,3,4]

[a] Department of Medical Education, Gundersen Lutheran Medical Foundation, 1900 South Avenue, C03-006A, La Crosse, WI 54601, USA
[b] Department of General and Vascular Surgery, Gundersen Lutheran Health System, 1900 South Avenue, C05-001, La Crosse, WI 54601, USA
* Corresponding author.
E-mail address: thcogbil@gundluth.org (T.H. Cogbill).

Surg Clin N Am 89 (2009) 727–738
doi:10.1016/j.suc.2009.02.005
0039-6109/09/$ – see front matter © 2009 Elsevier Inc. All rights reserved.
surgical.theclinics.com

Etiology

The exact etiology of MCC is not well understood, but several observations have been made. It seems to arise more frequently in sun-exposed areas of the body, although all areas have been described as primary sites. Perianal and vulvar sites have the worst prognosis of all primary sites. An increased incidence of MCC has been observed in patients who have HIV or cancer or have undergone organ transplant, suggesting a link between MCC and immunosuppression. Viral and carcinogenic chemical (eg, arsenic and methoxsalen) etiologies have been implied in the development of MCC. Numerous chromosomal abnormalities also have been observed, but a definitive causal relationship has not been established.

Presentation

MCC appears as a fast-growing, nontender, flesh- or red-blue–colored, firm intracu-taneous mass (**Fig. 1**). Most lesions are smaller than 2 cm in diameter at the time of diagnosis. MCC often arises in sun-exposed areas. Regional lymph nodes are involved in up to 30% of patients, and approximately 50% of patients develop systemic disease at some point. Secondary sites of spread include skin (28%), lymph nodes (27%), liver (13%), lung (10%), bone (10%), and brain (6%). Making the diagnosis of MCC clinically is difficult because the lesion can be mistaken for other cutaneous malignancies.[1,3]

Pathology

Histologic evaluation reveals a lesion that arises in the dermis and often extends into the subcutaneous tissue. The epidermis can be involved and may be ulcerated. The tumor consists of small blue cells with hyperchromatic nuclei and scant cytoplasm (**Fig. 2**). Mitoses, apoptosis, and lymphovascular invasion are common features. Three histologic subtypes have been described—intermediate, trabecular, and small cell—although no clinically significant differences have been described between subtypes. Immunohistochemical evaluation is necessary to distinguish MCC from other cancers. The pathologic differential diagnosis includes small-cell lung carcinoma, small-cell melanoma, lymphoma, and peripheral primitive neuroectodermal tumor.[1,3,4]

Evaluation and Staging

All patients with histologically confirmed MCC should undergo imaging to evaluate the extent of disease. Evaluation includes a thorough skin examination and chest

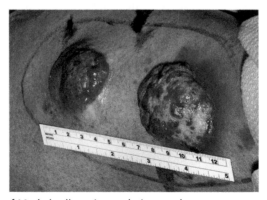

Fig. 1. Photograph of Merkel cell carcinoma lesions on leg.

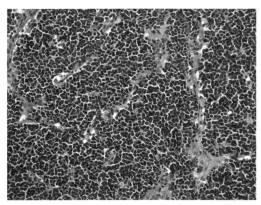

Fig. 2. Merkel cell carcinoma histology demonstrates sheets of cells with hyperchromatic nuclei and high nuclear-cytoplasmic ratio. The cells show characteristic nuclear molding and marked mitotic activity. (*Courtesy of* M. Arida, MD, and J. Janis, MD, La Crosse, WI.)

radiograph to exclude small-cell lung carcinoma. CT scans of the chest, abdomen, and pelvis are necessary to detect metastatic disease (**Fig. 3**). Head CT should be performed in symptomatic patients. Positron emission tomographic CT has been used in some studies in the evaluation of MCC and can be useful for staging and follow-up. Various staging systems based on size, nodal status, and metastasis have been proposed for MCC. The most recent system proposed by investigators at Memorial Sloan-Kettering is shown in **Table 1**.[1,5]

Treatment

Wide local excision (WLE) is the mainstay for treatment of disease that is confined to the skin. The degree of margin excision is not well defined, but 1- to 3-cm margins

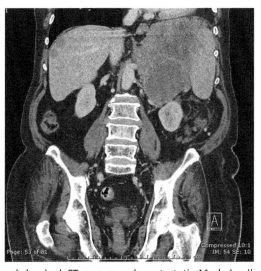

Fig. 3. Coronal view abdominal CT scan reveals metastatic Merkel cell carcinoma in large retroperitoneal mass and liver lesions.

Table 1 TNM staging for Merkel cell carcinoma	
Score	Characteristic
T1	Primary tumor < 2 cm in diameter
T2	Primary tumor $\geq$ 2 cm in diameter
N0	Negative regional lymph nodes
N1	Positive regional lymph nodes
M0	No distant metastatic disease
M1	Distant metastatic disease
Stage	TNM score combinations
I	T1, N0, M0
II	T2, N0, M0
III	Any T, N1, M0
IV	Any T, Any N, M1

Abbreviations: M, metastasis; N, node; T, tumor; TNM, tumor, node, metastasis.
Data from Allen PJ, Bowne WB, Jaques DP, et al. Merkel cell carcinoma: prognosis and treatment of patients from a single institution. J Clin Oncol 2005;23(10):2300–9.

have been recommended. In cosmetically sensitive areas, Mohs surgery may be help-ful, although research is limited.[1]

Lymph node dissection is often performed because up to one third of patients have nodal involvement. It is not clear whether lymph node dissection has an impact on survival, but it seems to benefit locoregional control. Clinically or radiographically posi-tive nodes should be resected, but it is unclear whether elective lymph node dissection provides benefit. Sentinel lymph node biopsy (SLNB) is a reasonable option in clini-cally node-negative patients to provide staging information and guide further treat-ment.[1,3,4] Nearly one third of patients who have MCC without clinical evidence of nodal disease have positive SLNB results.[6,7] In one study, 33% of patients with posi-tive SLNB results developed local, regional, or systemic recurrence of disease.[6] None of the 15 patients with positive SLNB results who underwent subsequent lymph node dissection experienced regional recurrence versus three of four patients in whom ther-apeutic lymphadenectomy was not performed. Gupta and associates[7] documented a 3-year recurrence rate of 60% in patients who had MCC and positive SLNB results versus 20% for patients with negative SLNB results. Patients with positive SLNB results who received additional treatment to the nodes had a relapse-free survival rate of 51% at 3 years versus 0% for patients who did not receive additional nodal therapy. Lymphadenectomy did not affect relapse-free survival rates in patients with negative SLNB results.[7]

MCC is a radiosensitive tumor, and radiation therapy is often used in combination with surgical excision, especially with positive or close excisional margins. Some have recommended routine postoperative radiation therapy to the primary tumor site for even localized disease.[4] Radiation therapy to the primary tumor site and regional lymph nodes can reduce locoregional recurrence rates, but the survival benefit is not known.[1]

Chemotherapy is used for nodal, metastatic, and recurrent MCC, but the optimal regimen is not established. The most common agents used are cyclophosphamide, anthracyclines, and cisplatin. Regimens are similar to those used for small-cell lung carcinoma. Response is seen in approximately 60% of patients. Because MCC is a disease that affects older patients, chemotherapy can be poorly tolerated secondary to associated comorbidities.[1,3,4]

Prognosis

The prognosis of MCC is related to the stage of disease. Five-year survival rate is 81% for stage I, 67% for stage II, 52% for stage III, and 11% for stage IV.[5] More than half of patients experience recurrence, usually within 1 year of treatment.[1,3]

Summary

MCC is an unusual, aggressive cutaneous malignancy that affects the elderly population but can be seen in younger, immunosuppressed patients. Disease confined to the skin is best managed by WLE. Multimodal treatment that consists of surgery, radiation, and chemotherapy is required for more widespread disease. Because of the rarity of recurrent or metastatic MCC, optimal treatment regimens have not yet been defined. Unfortunately, advanced disease and recurrence are common.

ECCRINE CARCINOMA

There are three types of sweat glands in the human body: eccrine, apocrine, and apoeccrine. Eccrine carcinoma is an extremely rare neoplasm of the eccrine sweat glands; it has a slow rate of growth and a high potential for recurrence. Numerous subtypes with different biologic and pathologic characteristics make the topic a challenging one. More than 10 subtypes are known, including eccrine porocarcinoma, hidradenocarcinoma, mucinous eccrine carcinoma, adenoid cystic carcinoma, aggressive digital papillary adenocarcinoma, microcystic adnexal carcinoma, mucoepidermoid carcinoma of the skin, eccrine spiradenoma, eccrine ductal adenocarcinoma, clear cell eccrine carcinoma, carcinosarcoma, and basaloid eccrine carcinoma.[8,9]

Epidemiology

Sweat gland malignancy accounts for approximately 0.005% of all malignant epithelial neoplasms.[8] In one series of 450,000 skin biopsy specimens, only 35 specimens were sweat gland carcinomas.[10] A review at the Mayo Clinic[8] covering more than 75 years of skin tumor specimens found 14 cases of eccrine carcinoma. Because of the rarity and the multiple subtypes, whether race or gender predisposes to the tumor is not well documented. Eccrine carcinoma occurs most often in patients over 50 years of age.

Etiology

The etiology is not known, but eccrine carcinoma can develop de novo from normal eccrine glands or from existing benign eccrine tumors. As with many other skin tumors, sunlight exposure and immunosuppression are thought to play a role.

Presentation

Most often these tumors present as a slow-growing, solitary, nontender, firm, nonulcerated dermal nodule that is fixed to the underlying tissue. The range of size at presentation in one series was 0.5 to 5 cm in diameter.[8] The most common sites of occurrence are the head, neck, and extremities, but various subtypes have unique distributions.[8–10]

Pathology

Because of the numerous subtypes and the varied appearance of each, a detailed histologic description of the subtypes is beyond the scope of this article; however, general characteristics include nuclear hyperchromasia, nuclear pleomorphism, nucleolar prominence, high nucleocytoplasmic ratios, and infiltration of vascular lumina (**Fig. 4**).[8] An experienced dermatopathologist is critical in the evaluation and management of these tumors because the differential diagnosis includes not only the various histologic subtypes but also a wide variety of other malignancies, including breast cancer, melanoma in situ, metastatic salivary gland cancer, metastatic gastrointestinal malignancies, clear cell thyroid cancer, Paget's disease, and Bowen's disease.[8] Numerous immunohistochemical stains are used to differentiate eccrine carcinoma from other malignancies and to differentiate subtypes. Definitive diagnosis with light microscopy alone is difficult.

Evaluation and Staging

A thorough history and physical examination are important in this rare malignancy because the differential diagnosis often includes metastatic skin deposits from other malignancies. Once the diagnosis has been confirmed by skin biopsy, further imaging studies may be needed, depending on the clinical scenario. Because of the rare nature of the disease, no specific recommendations regarding imaging can be made, but appropriate studies to exclude other metastatic primaries in the differential diagnosis should be performed. To the authors' knowledge, no specific staging criteria have been proposed.

Treatment

Surgical excision is the mainstay of treatment for this rare disease. Mohs surgery is advocated in many subtypes because they involve cosmetically sensitive areas and local recurrence is common.[8,10] In other areas, however, WLE or amputation (as in aggressive digital papillary adenocarcinoma) are the preferred treatments. Because of the rarity of this carcinoma, no specific recommendations regarding nodal dissection have been advanced. As a general rule, nodal metastasis from eccrine carcinoma is rare; nodal surgery is not likely to be necessary or beneficial in most cases.

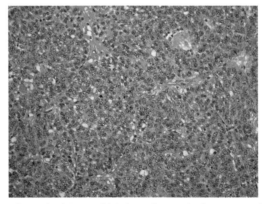

Fig. 4. Malignant eccrine spiradenoma histology demonstrates aggregates of basaloid cells with pleomorphic nuclei showing frequent mitotic activity. Scattered eccrine duct-like structures are visible. (*Courtesy of* M. Arida, MD, and J. Janis, MD, La Crosse, WI.)

No recommendations regarding the use of radiation or chemotherapy can be made, but treatment with either of these modalities should be considered as part of a multidisciplinary approach on a case-by-case basis. In a series from the Mayo Clinic, seven patients were treated with radiation and six experienced recurrence. The only patient treated with chemotherapy showed no clinical response. No survival benefit was found for either modality.[8]

Prognosis

Specific survival data are not known because of insufficient experience with these tumors. Metastasis is rare, except in certain subtypes that have more aggressive clinical behavior (such as aggressive digital papillary adenocarcinoma). Recurrence is common for all subtypes.[8–10]

Summary

Eccrine carcinoma is a rare sweat gland malignancy that is usually seen beyond the fifth decade of life. Diagnosis is difficult because the lesion is rare, has many subtypes, and is similar in appearance to metastatic cancer lesions. Treatment is based on complete surgical excision. Adjuvant therapies are poorly understood. Local recurrence is the rule, but metastases are uncommon except in certain subtypes. Chance of survival depends on subtype.

GLOMUS TUMORS

Glomus tumors (GTs) are uncommon neoplasms of the glomus body, an arteriovenous shunt in the skin that plays a role in temperature regulation. They were first described by Wood in 1812, and Masson later made the histologic diagnosis in 1924.[11] Glomus bodies are found throughout the skin but are concentrated in the digits. GTs are rarely malignant and can be solitary or multiple in presentation. Although glomus cells are found only in the skin, these rare tumors can have atypical extracutaneous locations.[12–15]

Epidemiology

The precise incidence of these rare tumors is unknown. In a review at the Mayo Clinic, GTs comprised only 1.6% of extremity soft tissue tumors.[15] Similarly, others have shown that GTs account for 1% to 4.5% of upper extremity tumors.[15] Men and women appear equally affected.[14–16] Age at presentation varies widely, with adults affected more often than children. Only 10% of GTs are multiple in presentation, and malignant GTs are rare, with only 45 cases described according to a 2005 review.[13,14]

Etiology

GTs are felt to arise from the glomus body by proliferation of one or more of its elements; however, the exact cause is unknown. Inherited patterns have been linked to defects in the glomin gene on chromosome 1.[12]

Presentation

Solitary and multiple variants of GTs exist. Most GTs are solitary in presentation and occur on the extremities, especially in the subungual area of the digits. The triad of hypersensitivity to cold, paroxysmal pain, and pinpoint pain suggests the diagnosis.[12] The lesions often have a bluish hue and are almost always smaller than 1 cm in diameter. Lesions larger than 1 cm suggest malignancy. Although digital locations are most common, GTs have been found in all parts of the body, including the viscera.[12,13,15] Multiple GTs are less often symptomatic.

Pathology

Histologically, GTs are irregularly shaped vascular spaces with compact nests of polygonal cells with round nuclei and eosinophilic cytoplasm (**Fig. 5**). Three benign histologic subtypes have been described, but the clinical relevance is unknown.[11] Solitary GTs are encapsulated, whereas the multiple variant is unencapsulated. Malignant GTs, also known as glomangiosarcomas, are characterized by large size (especially > 2 cm), deep location, atypical mitotic figures, moderate to high nuclear grade, large number of mitoses, and infiltrative growth.[16]

Evaluation

Most of these lesions are noticed because they are symptomatic, and clinical diagnosis can be made by the history and physical characteristics described previously. Three clinical tests have been described to help diagnose GTs. First, Love's test is performed by applying pressure precisely over the area of concern with a paperclip or pin. A positive test result produces severe pain and is reportedly 100% sensitive and 78% accurate. Second is Hildreth's test, in which a tourniquet is applied proximal to the lesion and Love's test is then performed. A positive test result should not produce pain. This is 71% sensitive and 78% accurate. Third, a cold sensitivity test shows increased pain with exposure to cold and was 100% sensitive and specific in a series of 18 patients.[12]

Further imaging with MRI can be performed if the diagnosis is elusive; however, its usefulness has been questioned.[12,13] In the case of malignant GTs, specific imaging guidelines have not been defined because of the small number of cases, with only 12 of 45 known cases having metastases.[14]

Treatment

Complete excision is recommended for solitary symptomatic lesions. For digital GTs, either a direct subungual or lateral digital incision can be used.[12] With the multiple variant, excision can be difficult secondary to the number of lesions. Alternative techniques, including sclerotherapy (with either hypertonic saline or sodium tetradecole-cylsulfate), electron beam radiation, and argon or carbon dioxide lasers, have been used.[13] Successful treatment of pulmonary metastases with chemotherapy has

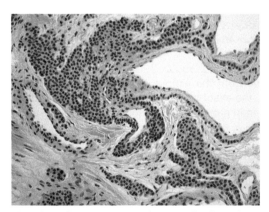

Fig. 5. Glomus tumor histology demonstrates uniform small cells with eosinophilic ctyoplasm associated with conspicuous vasculature. (*Courtesy of* M. Arida, MD, and J. Janis, MD, La Crosse, WI.)

been reported; however, because of the rarity of malignant GTs, the benefit of adjuvant treatments is uncertain.

Prognosis

Most GTs are benign, have no associated mortality, and rarely recur after local excision. Mortality is rare but has been documented in a handful of malignant cases.[13,16]

Summary

GTs are rare tumors that are usually painful, solitary, and located in the digits. Excision of solitary lesions is the recommended treatment, whereas multiple lesions may require alternative therapies. Recurrence, malignancy, and mortality are uncommon in these rare tumors.

DERMATOFIBROSARCOMA PROTUBERANS

First described in 1890, dermatofibrosarcoma protuberans (DFSP) is a rare soft tissue sarcoma that arises from the dermis. DFSP has an asymmetric growth pattern and tends to recur locally.[17–19] DFSP constitutes approximately 1% of all sarcomas and less than 0.1% of all malignancies.[19] Most (approximately 90%) are low-grade sarcomas, whereas the remainder are classified as intermediate grade because of a high-grade fibrosarcomatous component (DFSP-FS).[20]

Epidemiology

The annual incidence has been reported to be 4.2 per million. Blacks have a slightly higher incidence than whites; men and women are affected equally.[21] DFSP most commonly presents in the mid to late 30s; however, the disease can occur at any age.[17–19]

Etiology

The pathogenesis of DFSP is not completely understood. Some have associated its development with trauma, vaccinations, and scarring.[19] Recently, chromosomal abnormalities have been discovered, which suggest a genetic basis for this tumor. Translocation between chromosomes 17 and 22 has been observed in more than 90% of cases, resulting in the activation of platelet-derived growth factor receptor.[18]

Presentation

DFSP often presents as a solitary, asymptomatic, plaque-like cutaneous tumor that is violet to blue in color. The tumor usually exhibits slow growth and most commonly presents on the trunk, followed by the extremities, head, and neck. Most lesions are smaller than 5 cm in diameter, raised and firm, with surrounding telangiectasias. If untreated, the tumor can become noticeably protuberant.[17–19,22]

Pathology

Histologically, DFSP arises from the dermis as dense uniform cells that contain spindle-shaped nuclei. The cells are arranged into irregular interwoven fascicles in a storiform pattern, which is said to resemble a straw mat (**Fig. 6**). Tentacle-like projections of tumor are common, which may account for the high incidence of local recurrence after excision. Low- (DFSP) and intermediate-grade (DFSP-FS) variants exist. The "FS" denotes the high-grade fibrosarcomatous component present in this type, which constitutes approximately 10% of all cases.[17,19]

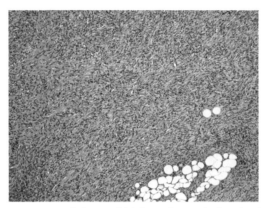

Fig. 6. Dermatofibrosarcoma protuberans histology demonstrates slender, uniform spindle cells with darkly staining nuclei and eosinophilic cytoplasm arrayed in a storiform pattern. Subcutaneous fat is entrapped by the tumor, resulting in a lace-like appearance. (*Courtesy of* M. Arida, MD, and J. Janis, MD, La Crosse, WI.)

Evaluation and Staging

Unless indicated by history and physical examination, extensive imaging is rarely needed because lymphatic or metastatic spread is uncommon. Suspicious lesions should undergo a core-needle, incisional, or excisonal biopsy to obtain histologic diagnosis. MRI can be used to determine the degree of local invasion and aid in surgical planning. If signs or symptoms of metastatic disease are present, further evaluation with CT or positron emission tomographic CT may be warranted.

Staging is made according to the American Musculoskeletal Tumor Society staging system, which is based on tumor grade and compartment involvement. Stage IA is a low-grade tumor confined to one tissue compartment, whereas stage IB extends into adjacent tissue compartments, that is, muscle or fascia. A stage II tumor by American Musculoskeletal Tumor Society definition is a high-grade lesion, and because DFSP is either low or intermediate grade, this distinction does not apply.[20]

Treatment

Surgical excision is the accepted treatment, although the type of surgery and width of surgical margins is a topic of debate. WLE with at least 3-cm margins has been the standard of care. Considerable variation of local recurrence from zero to more than 50% with WLE has been observed, which has led to the investigation of alternative techniques. In a recent series of 159 patients treated at Memorial Sloan-Kettering,[17] 21% of patients had a local recurrence, most of whom had close or positive margins. Mohs micrographic surgery has been shown to have excellent results with low rates of local recurrence.[18,19] The best role for Mohs micrographic surgery is likely in cosmetically sensitive areas. Some investigators advocate modified wide excision, a technique with Mohs-like horizontal sectioning of tissue, because this has been shown to have low rates of recurrence.[19] Although many techniques exist, WLE is the standard technique for DFSP in noncosmetically sensitive areas.

Treatment of positive or close margins should include re-excision, if possible. Radiation therapy has been used selectively in this instance if further surgery is not possible or would be cosmetically unacceptable, with good local control. Experience and data regarding radiation therapy are limited.[18,22,23] Metastatic disease is uncommon, but if isolated, surgical resection should be performed. Chemotherapeutic agents such as vinblastine and methotrexate have been used, but few data are available to make specific recommendations.[18] Because of DFSP tumor biology, imatinib, a platelet-derived growth factor receptor inhibitor, has been used with some success in advanced disease. In one series, 10 patients with locally advanced or metastatic disease were treated with imatinib, and all but 1 patient showed a response to treatment.[23]

Prognosis

Most patients with DFSP have an excellent outcome, despite the high recurrence rate. Metastatic disease is uncommon, occurring in only 1% to 2% of cases.[17,18] Mortality is also rare. In a series of 218 patients with DFSP, the 5- and 10-year mortality rates were 1.5% and 2.8%, respectively.[18] Based on a Memorial Sloan-Kettering study,[17] poor prognostic factors are (1) the DFSP-FS histologic subtype, (2) positive margins, (3) increased mitotic rate, (4) increased cellularity, and (5) age older than 50 years.

Summary

DFSP is a rare skin sarcoma characterized by local recurrence but low metastatic potential. Surgical WLE of primary and recurrent lesions is the mainstay of treatment. Additional therapies, such as radiation and imatinib administration, play a role in more aggressive disease.

ACKNOWLEDGMENTS

The authors gratefully acknowledge the contribution of Muammar Arida, MD, and John Janis, MD, from the Department of Pathology at Gundersen Lutheran Health System, who provided the four histology images.

REFERENCES

1. Goessling W, McKee PH, Mayer RJ. Merkel cell carcinoma. J Clin Oncol 2002; 20(2):588–98.
2. Toker C. Trabecular carcinoma of the skin. Arch Dermatol 1972;105(1):107–10.
3. Poulsen M. Merkel cell carcinoma of skin: diagnosis and management strategies. Drugs Aging 2005;22(3):219–29.
4. Poulsen M. Merkel-cell carcinoma of the skin. Lancet Oncol 2004;5(10):593–9.
5. Allen PJ, Bowne WB, Jaques DP, et al. Merkel cell carcinoma: prognosis and treatment of patients from a single institution. J Clin Oncol 2005;23(10):2300–9.
6. Mehrany K, Otley CC, Weenig RH, et al. A meta-analysis of the prognostic significance of sentinel lymph node status in Merkel cell carcinoma. Dermatol Surg 2002;28(2):113–7.
7. Gupta SG, Wang LC, Penas PF, et al. Sentinel lymph node biopsy for evaluation and treatment of patients with Merkel cell carcinoma: the Dana-Farber experience and meta-analysis of the literature. Arch Dermatol 2006;142(6):685–90.
8. Wick MR, Goellner JR, Wolfe JT 3rd, et al. Adnexal carcinomas of the skin. I. Eccrine carcinomas. Cancer 1985;56(5):1147–62.
9. Crowson AN, Magro CM, Mihm MC. Malignant adnexal neoplasms. Mod Pathol 2006;19(Suppl 2):S93–126.
10. Durairaj VD, Hink EM, Kahook MY, et al. Mucinous eccrine adenocarcinoma of the periocular region. Ophthal Plast Reconstr Surg 2006;22(1):30–5.
11. Tuncali D, Yilmaz AC, Terzioglu A, et al. Multiple occurrences of different histologic types of the glomus tumor. J Hand Surg [Am] 2005;30(1):161–4.

12. McDermott EM, Weiss AP. Glomus tumors. J Hand Surg [Am] 2006;31(8): 1397–400.
13. Parsons ME, Russo G, Fucich L, et al. Multiple glomus tumors. Int J Dermatol 1997;36(12):894–900.
14. Khoury T, Balos L, McGrath B, et al. Malignant glomus tumor: a case report and review of literature, focusing on its clinicopathologic features and immunohisto-chemical profile. Am J Dermatopathol 2005;27(5):428–31.
15. Schiefer TK, Parker WL, Anakwenze OA, et al. Extradigital glomus tumors: a 20-year experience. Mayo Clin Proc 2006;81(10):1337–44.
16. Folpe AL, Fanburg-Smith JC, Miettinen M, et al. Atypical and malignant glomus tumors: analysis of 52 cases, with a proposal for the reclassification of glomus tumors. Am J Surg Pathol 2001;25(1):1–12.
17. Bowne WB, Antonescu CR, Leung DH, et al. Dermatofibrosarcoma protuberans: a clinicopathologic analysis of patients treated and followed at a single institution. Cancer 2000;88(12):2711–20.
18. Fiore M, Miceli R, Mussi C, et al. Dermatofibrosarcoma protuberans treated at a single institution: a surgical disease with a high cure rate. J Clin Oncol 2005; 23(30):7669–75.
19. Yu W, Tsoukas MM, Chapman SM, et al. Surgical treatment for dermatofibrosar-coma protuberans: the Dartmouth experience and literature review. Ann Plast Surg 2008;60(3):288–93.
20. Dagan R, Morris CG, Zlotecki RA, et al. Radiotherapy in the treatment of derma-tofibrosarcoma protuberans. Am J Clin Oncol 2005;28(6):537–9.
21. Criscione VD, Weinstock MA. Descriptive epidemiology of dermatofibrosarcoma protuberans in the United States, 1973 to 2002. J Am Acad Dermatol 2007;56(6): 968–73.
22. Mendenhall WM, Zlotecki RA, Scarborough MT. Dermatofibrosarcoma protuber-ans. Cancer 2004;101(11):2503–8.
23. McArthur GA. Dermatofibrosarcoma protuberans: a surgical disease with a molecular savior. Curr Opin Oncol 2006;18(4):341–6.

Index

Note: Page numbers of article titles are in **boldface** type.

Surg Clin N Am 89 (2009) 739–746
doi:10.1016/S0039-6109(09)00053-X
0039-6109/09/$ – see front matter © 2009 Elsevier Inc. All rights reserved.

surgical.theclinics.com

Moving?

Make sure your subscription moves with you!

To notify us of your new address, find your **Clinics Account Number** (located on your mailing label above your name), and contact customer service at:

E-mail: elspcs@elsevier.com

800-654-2452 (subscribers in the U.S. & Canada)
314-453-7041 (subscribers outside of the U.S. & Canada)

Fax number: 314-523-5170

Elsevier Periodicals Customer Service
11830 Westline Industrial Drive
St. Louis, MO 63146

*To ensure uninterrupted delivery of your subscription, please notify us at least 4 weeks in advance of move.

Printed and bound by CPI Group (UK) Ltd, Croydon, CR0 4YY

03/10/2024

01040464-0018